THE EVERYDAY PALEO DIET COOKBOOK FOR BEGINNERS

YOUR ESSENTIAL GUIDE FOR EASY WEIGHT LOSS, REGULATE BLOOD SUGAR, REDUCE BODY INFLAMMATION AND ENJOY NUTRIENT-DENSE WHOLE FOODS RECIPES

CATHERINE JONES

Copyright Page

Table of Contents

CHAPTER 1: INTRODUCTION TO THE PALEO DIET

An understanding of the Paleo Diet's guiding concepts and background can be gained from reading the introduction. Fundamentally, the Paleo Diet seeks to replicate the prehistoric diets of our ancestors by emphasizing whole, unprocessed foods that were accessible in the Paleolithic period. This introduction to the diet explains its philosophy and emphasizes the eating of lean meats, fish, fruits, vegetables, nuts, and seeds; processed foods, grains, dairy products, and legumes are to be avoided. It explores the reasoning for this dietary strategy, referring to evolutionary biology and the idea that our bodies are more suited to the kinds of food that our ancestors once ate. Additionally, the introduction frequently discusses the possible health advantages of the Paleo Diet, including greater energy levels, weight control, and general health. In the conclusion, this part prepares readers to understand the underlying ideas and reasons for embracing a Paleo lifestyle.

Understanding the Core Principles

It is essential to comprehend the foundational ideas of the Paleo Diet in order to fully adopt its philosophy. This section explores the tenets that form the foundation of the diet in more detail. It clarifies the idea that our genetic composition is more in line with the eating habits of our prehistoric ancestors, who survived on readily available foods during the Paleolithic era. The necessity of eating complete, nutrient-dense foods is emphasized in this segment, along with the need to stay away from processed and refined foods that have become a part of modern agriculture and food processing.

Gaining an understanding of the underlying philosophy and scientific rationale of the Paleo Diet is essential to comprehending its fundamentals.

Paleolithic ancestral eating habits: The foundation of the Paleo diet is the theory that the meals that our Paleolithic ancestors ate are the ones that best suit our bodies. Hunter-gatherers at this time, people mostly ate entire, unprocessed foods such fish, lean meats, fruits, vegetables, nuts, and seeds. This time span comes before the agricultural revolution, which brought dairy, grains, and legumes into the human diet.

Whole foods & Nutrient Density: The fundamental idea places a strong emphasis on consuming nutrient-dense, whole foods. These meals provide the body with the most possible nutritional benefits because they are full of vital vitamins, minerals, and macronutrients in their natural state. They are unprocessed and devoid of artificial additives, supporting the theory that foods in their purest form are what our bodies are meant to eat.

Avoidance of Modern and Processed Foods: The Paleo Diet forgoes grains, vegetable oils, refined sugars, and processed foods. It is thought that these contemporary dietary changes to humans are a factor in a number of health concerns, including gastrointestinal disorders, insulin resistance, and inflammation. The diet seeks to lessen any potential negative impact certain foods may have on health by banning them.

Biological Adaptation and Evolutionary Biology: This dietary strategy contends that human genetics have not completely adjusted to the modifications brought about by contemporary agriculture and food processing, using evolutionary biology as support. It is thought that the foods that our ancestors ate for millions of years are genetically more suited to our bodies than the comparatively modern foods that have been added to the human diet in the last 10,000 years.

Health Benefits: Comprehending these fundamental ideas enables people to appreciate the possible health advantages of the Paleo diet. These could include better blood sugar regulation, decreased inflammation, better digestion, better weight management, and higher levels of energy.

By being aware of these concepts, people can choose their food more wisely and match their dietary practices more closely to the requirements that the human body has developed over eons of time. This knowledge serves as the cornerstone for people to make dietary choices that put their health and wellbeing first.

Historical Context and Evolution

To comprehend the Paleo Diet's tenets and reasoning, one must have a thorough awareness of its evolutionary background and historical context.

Paleolithic Period: The Paleo Diet is based on the Paleolithic Period, which lasted from roughly 2.5 million years ago to 10,000 years ago. Humans were mostly hunter-gatherers at this time, and they relied on meals found in their natural surroundings, including fruits, vegetables, nuts, seeds, wild game, and fish.

Shift to Agriculture: Humans made the switch from roving hunting and gathering communities to permanent farming communities some 10,000 years ago. With the advent of grains, legumes, and dairy farming during this agricultural revolution, the Paleolithic diet underwent a dramatic change.

Impact on Human Diet: When agriculture was introduced, the human diet changed to include items that had not previously played a major role in ancestral eating habits. Modern diets are based mostly on grains, legumes, and dairy, which became staples in many communities.

Evolutionary Adaptation: The Paleo Diet's proponents contend that the human body hasn't had enough time to genetically adjust to these relatively recent nutritional modifications brought about by agriculture. They contend that the diets of the Paleolithic epoch still have a greater influence on our genetic make-up.

Modern diet vs. Ancient Diet: The historical background draws attention to the differences between the diet that humans have evolved to eat over millions of years and the diet that is popular in the present era, which is defined by processed foods, refined sweets, and a large amount of grains and dairy products.

This historical evolution of human dietary patterns lays the groundwork for the Paleo Diet, which holds that going back to a diet more like that of our prehistoric ancestors may better meet the nutritional requirements of the human body and may even provide health benefits by avoiding foods that were introduced after agriculture.

CHAPTER 2: THE SCIENCE AND BENEFITS OF PALEO

Exploring the scientific foundations and possible health and well-being benefits of the Paleo Diet is essential to understanding its science and benefits. Fundamentally, the diet is based on an evolutionary viewpoint, implying that our genetic composition is closer to that of our Paleolithic predecessors. Whole, unprocessed foods like lean meats, fish, fruits, vegetables, nuts, and seeds made up the majority of this traditional diet. It is believed that a return to a more ancestral style of eating is necessary since our bodies may not have fully acclimated to the nutritional changes brought about by modern agriculture and food processing.

The concept that complete, nutrient-dense diets offer vital vitamins, minerals, and macronutrients necessary for optimum health is supported by scientific study. These meals may have a number of health advantages since they frequently lack the processed ingredients, preservatives, and additives seen in many modern diets. The Paleo Diet's emphasis on avoiding refined carbohydrates, artificial additives, and processed foods is in line with scientific findings that relate these items' excessive intake to inflammation, obesity, insulin resistance, and a host of chronic conditions.

Additionally, research and firsthand accounts link the Paleo Diet to a number of health advantages. Enhanced cardiovascular health, less inflammation, better blood sugar regulation, better weight management, and improved digestive function are a few of these. It may be useful in treating diseases including type 2 diabetes and metabolic syndrome, according to some research. To properly evaluate the diet's benefits on long-term health outcomes, more thorough and long-term study across varied groups is necessary, even though the studies that are already available show promise.

Comprehending the scientific foundation and substantiation of the Paleo Diet enables folks to make knowledgeable decisions regarding their eating patterns. It draws attention to the possible benefits of eating entire, unprocessed foods instead of refined and processed goods. However, further investigation is still necessary to clarify the diet's wider effects on many health indicators and its long-term viability as a nutritional strategy.

Scientific Basis and Evolutionary Perspective

Drawing from the "Scientific Basis and Evolutionary Perspective," the Paleo Diet seeks to replicate the eating habits of our prehistoric predecessors, particularly those of the Paleolithic era, on the theory that our bodies were better suited to the foods that were consumed at that time. The foundation of this dietary strategy is based on some ideas that are consistent with evolutionary theories of human nutrition.

Hunter-Gatherer Lifestyle: The Paleo Diet, which mostly consists of lean meats, fish, fruits, vegetables, nuts, and seeds, is inspired by the diet that our hunter-gatherer ancestors are thought to have followed. The argument is that these are the foods that our bodies were designed to digest well over time.

Evolutionary Adaptation: Proponents contend that there hasn't been much genetic evolution since the Paleolithic era, implying that our bodies may have evolved to be more adapted to the diets that were available then rather than the processed foods of today.

Nutrient Density and the Removal of Processed Foods: Whole, unprocessed foods that are high in nutrients and devoid of refined sugars, additives, and preservatives are prioritized. The goal of this strategy is to give a diet that is higher in nutrients and more like what our predecessors ate.

Avoidance of Grains and Legumes: Because these foods were not commonly consumed during the Paleolithic era, the diet excludes grains, legumes, and dairy products. Proponents claim that because certain foods may include allergies or anti-nutrients, they could have a negative impact on one's health.

Emphasis on High-Quality Protein and Healthy Fats: The Paleo diet frequently places a premium on high-quality protein sources, such fish that is caught in the wild and grass-fed meats, and it also promotes the use of healthy fats from foods like avocados, almonds, and olive oil.

Potential Health Benefits: According to some research, following a Paleo-style diet may help with blood sugar regulation, weight loss, and general health markers. Science is still studying the long-term impacts and overall health results, though.

Although the Paleo Diet is consistent with the evolutionary theory of human food history, it is important to remember that the idea of replicating prehistoric diets has its detractors:

- Lack of Complete Understanding: There are still questions regarding the precise makeup of prehistoric diets because our knowledge of Paleolithic meals is dependent on conjecture and archaeological data.

- Variation in Human Evolution: It is challenging to identify a universal "Paleo Diet" because human groups in different places have varied diets depending on available resources.

- Limited study and Long-Term consequences: Individual responses to such dietary patterns may vary, and study is still needed to determine the long-term consequences and possible health hazards of rigidly adhering to a Paleo diet.

In summary, the Paleo Diet proposes that our bodies may be well suited to particular foods eaten during the Paleolithic epoch by integrating an evolutionary viewpoint on human nutrition. It encourages entire, nutrient-dense foods, but more research is need to completely understand its long-term effects on health because of its tight standards and exclusions, which may not be suitable for everyone.

Health Benefits and Positive Effects

Drawing on its ideas rooted in evolutionary perspectives on nutrition, the Paleo Diet has gained attention for a number of reasons and is frequently linked to beneficial health outcomes. Here are a few alleged health advantages and favorable outcomes that the Paleo diet is frequently linked to:

Weight Loss: Proponents contend that by fostering satiety and naturally lowering calorie consumption, the Paleo Diet's emphasis on whole, unprocessed foods, lean proteins, and healthy fats can aid in weight loss.

Better Blood Sugar Control: People with diabetes or insulin resistance may benefit from the Paleo Diet's ability to better control blood sugar levels by avoiding processed carbohydrates and refined sugars.

Increased Nutrient consumption: Eating more fresh fruits, vegetables, lean meats, and nuts can lead to an increase in the consumption of vital nutrients that are good for your body in general, such as vitamins, minerals, and antioxidants.

Improved Digestive Health: Removing grains and legumes, which include substances like lectins and phytates that can upset some people's stomachs, may help some people's digestive systems.

Decreased Inflammation: According to some supporters, focusing on whole, anti-inflammatory foods instead of processed meals may help lower chronic inflammation in the body, which may be beneficial for a number of inflammatory-related health disorders.

Possibility of Allergy and Sensitivity Reduction: Reducing certain food groups, such as dairy or wheat, may help people with certain food allergies or sensitivities feel better.

Support for a Healthy Microbiome: Eating more fruits and vegetables high in fiber can improve gut health and foster a varied, balanced microbiome that is related to general wellbeing.

Promotion of Satiety and Energy Levels: The Paleo Diet's greater protein and healthy fat intake may encourage feelings of fullness and sustained energy, which may help to improve energy levels throughout the day and maybe lessen cravings.

CHAPTER 3: PALEO DIET FOOD GUIDELINES

The Paleo Diet is based on an evolutionary theory of human nutrition and consists of eating foods that are thought to have been consumed by our Paleolithic ancestors. The focus of this dietary strategy is on entire, unadulterated foods that early humans may have fished or hunted. It emphasizes a range of fruits and vegetables, nuts, seeds, avocados, olive oil, and healthy fats like those in nuts and seeds, as well as lean proteins like wild-caught fish and grass-fed meats. The diet's opponents argue that because of its composition or contemporary processing techniques, grains, legumes, processed foods, refined sugars, and the majority of dairy products may have negative health impacts. These items were not a component of the diet of our ancestors.

Paleo Diet proponents assert that the diet may help with weight loss, better blood sugar regulation, higher nutritional intake, enhanced gut health, less inflammation, and support for a balanced gut microbiota, among other possible health advantages. The rigorous rules of the diet, however, might not be suitable for everyone, and there is continuous discussion about its long-term viability and possible nutrient shortages as a result of the elimination of whole food groups.

People's reactions to the Paleo diet might differ greatly, therefore it's important for each person to take into account their own health requirements, preferences, and possible deviations. It is advisable to get advice from healthcare specialists or trained dietitians prior to implementing substantial dietary modifications to guarantee adequate nutrition and alignment with personal health objectives. Even though the Paleo Diet is inspired by evolutionary theory, it should be applied with a balanced awareness of both its advantages and disadvantages.

Approved Foods List and Benefits

Lean Proteins: Include Seafood, fish, and meats raised on grass. These protein sources are high in vital elements that promote overall health, brain function, and muscle health, such as iron, zinc, and omega-3 fatty acids.

Vegetables and Fruits: Promotes the intake of a broad range of fruits and vegetables, which include a number of antioxidants, fiber, vitamins, and minerals. They lower the chance of developing chronic illnesses, enhance healthy digestion, and improve immune function.

Nuts and Seeds: Nuts and seeds such as flaxseeds, walnuts, and almonds are excellent providers of protein, healthy fats, and a range of vitamins and minerals. They are high in energy, have anti-inflammatory qualities, and support heart health.

Heart-healthy, brain-functioning, and energy-boosting monounsaturated and saturated fats are found in avocados, olive oil, coconut oil, and lipids from grass-fed animals.

These authorized meals provide the following advantages:

Weight control: Because whole, unprocessed foods are lower in empty calories and more satisfying, they help with weight management by encouraging satiety.

Increased Nutrient Intake: Foods high in vitamins, minerals, antioxidants, and healthy fats, such as fruits, vegetables, nuts, and lean proteins, promote general health and wellbeing.

Stabilized Blood Sugar: The Paleo Diet may help control blood sugar levels by avoiding refined carbs and processed sweets, which may be advantageous for those who have diabetes or insulin sensitivity.

Decreased Inflammation: By emphasizing whole, anti-inflammatory foods, the diet may help lower chronic inflammation, which is linked to a number of health problems, such as autoimmune disorders and heart disease.

Better Digestive Health: For some people, removing some potentially irritating food groups (such as grains and legumes) may help with better digestion.

While there are many health benefits associated with these Paleo Diet-approved meals, it's important to keep a balanced view that takes individual needs and potential variances into account. To further maximize the health benefits of the diet while addressing personal health goals, make sure you are getting a well-rounded intake of nutrients and seek advice from medical specialists or registered dietitians.

Foods to Avoid and Their Impact

Some items are usually avoided in the Paleo Diet because they are not included in the assumed ancient diet. Below is a list of foods that are frequently off-limits on the Paleo diet along with possible side effects:

Grains: Certain people may have trouble digesting gluten and other substances found in wheat, barley, oats, and other grains. Proponents contend that they can induce inflammation in the body and that they may aggravate digestive problems including bloating or pain.

Legumes: Beans, lentils, peanuts, and soybeans include substances called lectins and phytates that, according to some, may prevent certain people from absorbing nutrients properly and may also upset their digestive systems.

Dairy Products: Because of its lactose content (milk sugar) and the idea that humans did not eat dairy during the Paleolithic era, milk, cheese, yogurt, and other dairy products are not allowed on the Paleo diet. Some people have an intolerance to lactose, which can cause gas, bloating, and diarrhea.

Processed Foods and Refined Sugars: Due to their lack of nutritional content and possible detrimental health effects, such as influencing blood sugar levels and causing weight gain, highly processed foods, refined sugars, artificial sweeteners, and additives should be avoided.

Refined Vegetable Oils: Because of their high omega-6 fatty acid concentration, oils including corn oil, soybean oil, and sunflower oil are not included. An excessive ratio of omega-6 to omega-3 in the diet can aggravate inflammation and lead to a number of health problems.

The Paleo diet's effects of eliminating these foods are frequently linked to possible health advantages:

Better Digestive Health: Removing grains and legumes can help some people feel better about their digestive systems and create a more favorable environment in the stomach.

Potential Weight Management: By limiting the consumption of empty calories and encouraging a diet high in whole, nutrient-dense foods, avoiding processed foods and refined sugars may help with weight management.

Decreased Inflammation: Eliminating specific foods that are thought to aggravate inflammation may cause the body's inflammatory response to decrease, which may help people who suffer from inflammatory diseases.

Blood Sugar Regulation: Reducing processed carbs and refined sugars may help control blood sugar levels, which may be advantageous for those who have diabetes or insulin resistance.

It's crucial to remember that different people may react differently to the elimination of certain meals. Research on the long-term consequences of strictly adhering to the Paleo Diet is still ongoing, and some people may not see significant advantages. A well-rounded nutritional intake should be prioritized, and speaking with medical specialists or registered dietitians can assist people in making dietary decisions that are tailored to their own requirements and objectives.

CHAPTER 4: IMPLEMENTING THE PALEO DIET

There are a number of critical procedures that must be followed in order to adhere to the concepts and standards of the Paleo Diet. Get to know the permitted foods first. These include lean proteins (such as grass-fed beef and wild-caught fish), a variety of veggies and fruits, nuts, seeds, and healthy fats (such as olive oil and avocados). In order to plan meals and buy for groceries, it is necessary to have an understanding of these permitted food groups.

Restrictions on grains, legumes, processed foods, refined sugars, and the majority of dairy products must thereafter be removed from the diet. In order to stay on track with the diet, it may be necessary to read labels and pay attention to the components in packaged meals. As part of the change, it's common to replace certain pantry staples with others that have been authorized.

Following the Paleo Diet requires meticulous meal preparation. In order to maintain a healthy diet and achieve nutritional balance, it is helpful to create meal plans that include a range of allowed foods. To get maximum taste without depending on restricted ingredients, it is necessary to experiment with new recipes, use varied fruits and vegetables, and explore alternate cooking methods.

In addition, it is critical to keep an eye on food quality. Following the diet's recommendation of eating only whole, unprocessed foods means giving preference to organic, grass-fed, and sustainably sourced products whenever feasible. In keeping with the diet's tenets, it is recommended that you shop for meat, fish, and vegetables at local farmers' markets or from other reputable sources.

When you're on the Paleo Diet, it might be difficult to adjust to social circumstances and eat out. Hosts and restaurant employees can better meet guests' requirements if they are informed in advance of any food allergies or limitations. To stay on track with the plan when eating out, stick to lighter fare like lean meats and veggies, and cut out the dairy and grains.

Lastly, it is reasonable to expect most people to be flexible and allow for rare departures from the stringent rules. While maintaining a consistent eating plan is essential, it's possible to make small concessions here and there to accommodate cravings or celebrate special occasions without completely abandoning the diet's guiding principles.

Understanding the Paleo Diet's principles, meal planning, making educated food choices, and tailoring the diet to personal preferences and situations are all crucial for a successful implementation. To get the possible benefits of this eating plan, adaptability and an emphasis on whole, nutrient-dense meals are key.

Transition Strategies and Preparation

If you want to successfully adopt the principles of the Paleo Diet, you need to prepare ahead of time and make little changes. Learning the basics of the diet, such as the allowed and prohibited food groups, is a good place to start. With this information in hand, a more seamless change may be accomplished. To make the transition easier and less disruptive to your diet, try cutting back on banned items and adding in more allowed alternatives little by little.

When starting the Paleo Diet, it is essential to plan ahead for your meals. The best way to start is to eat more Paleo-friendly meals, try out new recipes, and cut out non-compliant items one by one. By making sure Paleo-friendly alternatives are on hand and minimizing the need to resort to non-compliant items when time is of the essence, meal preparing for the week may make compliance easier.

To make room for Paleo, purge the fridge and pantry of anything that isn't part of the diet. Swapping out these goods for diet-approved substitutes makes sticking to the plan easier and less tempting. Make sure you have an abundance of recommended foods on hand by stocking up on lean meats, produce, nuts, and healthy fats.

During this time of change, it might be helpful to reach out for assistance. You can get helpful hints, recipes, and support from others who are already on the Paleo Diet if you join an online community or ask for advice from those who have been there. For more ideas and information, try looking for Paleo-friendly recipes in cookbooks, on blogs, or in social media.

The Paleo Diet can be more easily and sustainably implemented with little tweaks and modifications along the way rather than a complete overhaul. Another way to make the change easier, avoid cravings, and stick to the plan for the long haul is to be flexible and allow for occasional treats. Making a smooth transition to and staying on the Paleo Diet is possible with the right amount of planning, information, slow progress, and support.

Meal Planning and Recipes

While following the Paleo Diet, it is important to avoid grains, legumes, processed foods, and the majority of dairy products while planning meals. Instead, focus on creating balanced meals that are high in permitted foods. A good starting point is to base meals on lean proteins such as eggs, grass-fed beef, chicken, and fish. Incorporating a rainbow of fruits and vegetables into your protein-rich diet guarantees a wide range of minerals, vitamins, and antioxidants. Avocados, almonds, seeds, and olive oil are good sources of healthy fats that can help you feel full and satisfied after eating.

To save time and make sure you always have Paleo-friendly alternatives on hand, it's a good idea to make a weekly meal plan. Meal planning becomes much easier when you focus on protein sources and supplement them with veggies and healthy fats. An easy-to-make Paleo dinner may be grilled chicken with roasted veggies and a dab of olive oil, or it could be a salad of salmon, mixed greens, and avocado.

Finding Paleo-friendly recipes is essential for keeping meals interesting and varied. Cookbooks, websites, and social media sites that only provide Paleo recipes are just a few of the many options out there. If you're looking for a grain-free side dish to go with your main course, try these recipes: cauliflower rice, zucchini noodles, or sweet potato fries. To keep to the Paleo diet's principals while still enjoying some of your favorite foods, try making cauliflower pizza crust, lettuce wrap tacos, or pancakes with coconut flour.

Preparing meals in advance and cooking in bulk might be helpful for people with hectic schedules. Make sure you have plenty of Paleo-friendly meals to eat all week long by making a big batch of them and keeping them in portions. To make healthy meals quickly and with little mess, try using a slow cooker, an Instant Pot, or a one-pan recipe.

Without resorting to manufactured foods, Paleo meals may be flavorfully enhanced by experimenting with various herbs, spices, and seasonings. Spices, fresh herbs, ginger, turmeric, and garlic all contribute flavor without deviating from the diet.

At its core, the Paleo Diet is all about variety and creativity when it comes to meal preparation. It's about finding the right combination of meats, veggies, fruits, and healthy fats. Meal prepping and using one of the many Paleo-friendly recipes may make sticking to the diet easier without sacrificing flavor or nutrition.

CHAPTER 5: PALEO DIET FOR HEALTH AND WELLNESS

Many people believe that the Paleo Diet, which forgoes manufactured meals in favor of full, nutrient-dense ones, may improve their health and well-being. The fact that it may help with weight management is a major plus. The diet may help with weight reduction or maintenance by emphasizing whole foods that are high in protein and good fats, which may lead to a decrease in calorie consumption and an increase in fullness.

Also, better control of blood sugar levels may result from the diet's emphasis on whole, low-glycemic foods and the avoidance of processed carbs and refined sugars. People trying to control their blood sugar levels or who suffer from diabetes may find this feature very helpful.

There are some who think that the elimination of processed foods, grains, and legumes from the Paleo Diet helps bring down inflammation levels. More study is required in this area, although following an anti-inflammatory diet like the Paleo Diet may have possible advantages for inflammation-related disorders and the many health problems that are linked to chronic inflammation.

Fruits, vegetables, nuts, and seeds are examples of nutrient-rich foods that are eaten in their entire form. These foods include important vitamins, minerals, antioxidants, and good fats, which contribute to general wellness. There is some evidence that eating these foods can help with digestion, immunity, and preventing chronic illnesses.

Despite the Paleo Diet's advocates and its advantages, it's important to recognize the diet's possible drawbacks and the fact that everyone is different. Without proper preparation, vitamin deficiencies might result from cutting out whole food categories like grains and dairy. The scientific community is still debating and researching the long-term consequences and sustainability of the Paleo Diet.

When contemplating the Paleo Diet for health and wellbeing, it's important to keep in mind that everyone's needs, interests, and circumstances are different. Individuals can benefit from meeting their nutritional demands in a way that is consistent with their health objectives by consulting with healthcare providers or certified dietitians before making any dietary decisions.

Weight Management and Improved Energy

By eliminating manufactured meals in favor of whole, nutrient-dense ones, the Paleo Diet helps people maintain a healthy weight. Refined sweets and processed carbs are automatically reduced on this diet because lean proteins, healthy fats, and an abundance of veggies and fruits take center stage. This composition is great for those who are trying to lose weight or keep the weight off since it makes you feel full on less calories. By putting an emphasis on whole, unprocessed meals, you may control your hunger and maybe avoid the overeating that comes with processed foods.

Additionally, the elimination of processed carbs and refined sugars from the Paleo Diet contributes to the maintenance of healthy blood sugar levels. Improved energy stability all day long is a result of this stabilization, which lessens the ebb and flow of energy that follows high-glycemic meal consumption. The diet helps maintain steady energy levels without the peaks and valleys caused by fast carbohydrate consumption, which comes mostly from fruits and vegetables, along with healthy fats and proteins.

A key component of the Paleo Diet's success in weight loss and energy enhancement is its focus on protein and healthy fats. The regulation of metabolism and weight can be aided by consuming protein-rich meals, which also contribute to feelings of fullness and the preservation of muscle mass. Also, a concentrated source of energy, the good fats found in foods like almonds, avocados, and olive oil can keep you mentally and physically active for a long time.

Nonetheless, it's crucial to tackle weight loss and increased energy levels taking into account individual differences and lifestyle choices in general. when many people may find success with these objectives when following the Paleo Diet, results may vary greatly depending on variables including metabolic rate, degree of physical activity, and general health. Sustainable weight control and enhanced energy levels may be achieved through a balanced strategy that takes into account individual requirements and preferences, in addition to regular physical exercise and enough sleep. You may get individualized advice on how to include the Paleo Diet into a comprehensive plan for weight loss and energy improvement by consulting with healthcare experts or certified dietitians.

Enhanced Nutritional Intake and Digestive Health

Improved dietary intake is largely attributable to the Paleo Diet's focus on whole, nutrient-dense meals. The diet supplies a wide range of macronutrients, antioxidants, vitamins, and minerals by emphasizing a diversity of produce, lean meats, nuts, seeds, and healthy fats. Because of the wide variety of phytochemicals and minerals it contains, this nutritional treasure trove promotes health and wellness on all levels.

The Paleo Diet promotes intestinal health and better nutrient absorption by eating enough of fruits and vegetables. Due to their high fiber content, these plant-based meals support good digestion and intestinal flora. Constipation and diverticulitis are two digestive disorders that fiber can help prevent by regulating bowel motions and encouraging the growth of good bacteria in the gut. In addition, there is some evidence that the phytochemicals and antioxidants included in produce can help keep the digestive system healthy and lessen inflammation.

Moreover, for some people, the elimination of processed foods, refined carbohydrates, and additives from the Paleo Diet may help with gastrointestinal issues. Some people experience gastrointestinal distress after consuming processed foods due to the presence of artificial chemicals and preservatives. The diet promotes a healthy gut environment by limiting the use of processed meals and increasing the consumption of whole, unprocessed foods.

Although there may be noticeable improvements to digestive health and a focus on natural foods on the Paleo Diet, results may vary from person to person. While some may see an improvement in their gastrointestinal symptoms, others may not notice any difference at all. A balanced intake of nutrients is also critical, as is taking into account individual demands and differences. For individualized advice on how to maximize nutrient intake and promote digestive health while following the Paleo Diet or any diet plan, it's a good idea to consult with healthcare providers or certified dietitians.

CHAPTER 6: NUTRIENT-DENSE, WHOLE FOODS PALEO DIET RECIPES

PALEO DIET BREAKFAST RECIPES

Vegetable Frittata

Ingredients:

6 eggs

1/4 cup almond milk or coconut milk

1 tablespoon olive oil or coconut oil

1 small onion, diced

1 bell pepper, diced

1 cup spinach, chopped

1 tomato, diced

Salt and pepper to taste

Fresh herbs (such as parsley or basil), chopped (optional)

Instructions:

Preheat your oven to 350°F (175°C).

In a bowl, whisk together the eggs, almond or coconut milk, salt, and pepper until well combined. Set aside.

Heat olive oil or coconut oil in an oven-safe skillet over medium heat.

Add diced onion and bell pepper to the skillet and sauté for 3-4 minutes until they start to soften.

Add chopped spinach to the skillet and cook for an additional 1-2 minutes until wilted.

Pour the egg mixture evenly over the sautéed vegetables in the skillet.

Add diced tomatoes on top of the egg mixture.

Cook on the stovetop for about 3-4 minutes until the edges start to set.

Transfer the skillet to the preheated oven and bake for 12-15 minutes or until the frittata is fully set and slightly golden on top.

Once done, remove the skillet from the oven and let it cool for a few minutes.

Slice the frittata into wedges, garnish with fresh herbs if desired, and serve warm.

Paleo Banana Pancakes

Ingredients:

2 ripe bananas

4 eggs

1/2 teaspoon cinnamon

1/4 teaspoon vanilla extract (optional)

Coconut oil for cooking

Instructions:

In a mixing bowl, mash the ripe bananas with a fork until smooth.

Add the eggs, cinnamon, and vanilla extract (if using) to the mashed bananas. Whisk everything together until well combined.

Heat a skillet or griddle over medium heat and lightly grease it with coconut oil.

Pour small amounts of the pancake batter onto the skillet to form pancakes.

Cook for about 2-3 minutes on each side until golden brown, flipping carefully.

Once cooked, remove the pancakes from the skillet and continue cooking the remaining batter.

Serve the Paleo Banana Pancakes warm with a drizzle of honey or a sprinkle of fresh fruit for added sweetness, if desired.

Paleo Chia Seed Breakfast Bowl

Ingredients:

1/4 cup chia seeds

1 cup almond milk or coconut milk

1/2 teaspoon vanilla extract

1 tablespoon honey or maple syrup (optional)

Mixed berries (such as strawberries, blueberries, raspberries)

Sliced almonds or chopped nuts (optional)

Unsweetened shredded coconut (optional)

Instructions:

In a bowl or container, mix the chia seeds, almond milk (or coconut milk), vanilla extract, and honey or maple syrup (if using). Stir well to combine.

Let the mixture sit in the refrigerator for at least 2 hours or overnight, allowing the chia seeds to absorb the liquid and form a pudding-like consistency.

Once the chia seed pudding has set, remove it from the refrigerator.

Top the pudding with a generous amount of mixed berries.

Optionally, sprinkle sliced almonds or chopped nuts for added crunch and unsweetened shredded coconut for extra flavor and texture.

Serve the Paleo Chia Seed Breakfast Bowl chilled and enjoy this nutritious and flavorful breakfast packed with antioxidants, fiber, and healthy fats.

Paleo Avocado Egg Cups

Ingredients:

2 ripe avocados

4 eggs

Salt and pepper to taste

Chopped fresh herbs (optional, for garnish)

Instructions:

Preheat the oven to 425°F (220°C).

Cut the avocados in half and remove the pits. Scoop out a little extra avocado flesh from each half to create a larger hollow for the egg.

Place the avocado halves on a baking dish, ensuring they are stable and won't tip over.

Crack one egg into each avocado half, making sure it fits within the hollow and doesn't overflow.

Sprinkle salt and pepper on top of each egg.

Bake in the preheated oven for about 15-20 minutes, or until the egg whites are set and the yolks reach your desired level of doneness.

Once done, remove the avocado egg cups from the oven.

Garnish with chopped fresh herbs if desired, and serve these delicious and creamy Paleo Avocado Egg Cups warm.

Paleo Breakfast Skillet

Ingredients:

4 slices of bacon, chopped

1 sweet potato, peeled and diced

1 bell pepper, diced

1 small onion, diced

2 cloves garlic, minced

4 eggs

Salt and pepper to taste

Fresh parsley or cilantro for garnish (optional)

Instructions:

In a skillet over medium heat, cook the chopped bacon until it becomes crispy. Remove the bacon from the skillet and set it aside, leaving the rendered fat in the skillet.

Add diced sweet potato to the skillet with the rendered bacon fat. Cook for about 5-7 minutes, stirring occasionally, until the sweet potatoes start to soften.

Add diced bell pepper and onion to the skillet. Cook for an additional 5 minutes until the vegetables are tender.

Add minced garlic to the skillet and cook for 1-2 minutes until fragrant.

Return the crispy bacon to the skillet and mix it with the vegetables.

Create small wells in the mixture for the eggs.

Crack eggs into the wells. Cover the skillet and cook until the eggs are set to your desired level (about 5-7 minutes for runny yolks).

Season with salt and pepper to taste.

Garnish with fresh parsley or cilantro if desired and serve this hearty Paleo Breakfast Skillet warm.

Paleo Sausage and Veggie Breakfast Casserole

Ingredients:

1 pound ground breakfast sausage (look for sugar-free or Paleo-friendly)

1 onion, diced

1 bell pepper, diced

2 cups spinach, chopped

8 eggs

1/4 cup coconut milk or almond milk

Salt and pepper to taste

Cooking fat (coconut oil, ghee, or olive oil)

Instructions:

Preheat the oven to 375°F (190°C).

In a skillet over medium heat, cook the ground sausage until browned. Remove the cooked sausage from the skillet and set it aside.

In the same skillet, add diced onion and bell pepper. Cook for about 3-4 minutes until they start to soften.

Add chopped spinach to the skillet and cook for an additional 1-2 minutes until wilted. Remove the skillet from heat.

In a mixing bowl, whisk together the eggs, coconut milk or almond milk, salt, and pepper until well combined.

Grease a baking dish with cooking fat.

Spread the cooked sausage evenly on the bottom of the baking dish.

Top the sausage with the cooked vegetables from the skillet.

Pour the egg mixture over the sausage and vegetables in the baking dish.

Bake in the preheated oven for 25-30 minutes or until the eggs are set and the top is lightly golden.

Once done, remove the casserole from the oven and let it cool for a few minutes.

Slice and serve this flavorful and protein-packed Paleo Sausage and Veggie Breakfast Casserole for a delightful morning meal.

Paleo Spinach and Mushroom Omelette

Ingredients:

3 eggs

1 cup fresh spinach leaves, chopped

1/2 cup mushrooms, sliced

1/4 cup diced onion

1 tablespoon coconut oil or ghee

Salt and pepper to taste

Optional: diced tomatoes, avocado slices, or fresh herbs for garnish

Instructions:

In a bowl, whisk the eggs until well beaten. Season with salt and pepper.

Heat coconut oil or ghee in a skillet over medium heat.

Add diced onion and sliced mushrooms to the skillet. Cook for about 3-4 minutes until the mushrooms start to brown and the onions become translucent.

Add chopped spinach to the skillet and cook for an additional 1-2 minutes until the spinach wilts.

Pour the beaten eggs over the cooked vegetables in the skillet, ensuring an even distribution.

Allow the eggs to cook for a couple of minutes until the edges begin to set.

Gently lift the edges of the omelette with a spatula and tilt the skillet to let the uncooked egg flow to the edges.

Once the omelette is mostly set but still slightly runny on top, carefully fold it in half using the spatula.

Cook for another minute or until the eggs are fully cooked through.

Slide the omelette onto a plate, garnish with diced tomatoes, avocado slices, or fresh herbs if desired, and serve this wholesome and nutritious Paleo Spinach and Mushroom Omelette while warm.

Paleo Breakfast Smoothie Bowl

Ingredients:

1 frozen banana, sliced

1/2 cup mixed berries (such as strawberries, blueberries, raspberries)

1/2 cup coconut milk or almond milk

1 tablespoon almond butter or cashew butter

Toppings: sliced almonds, shredded coconut, chia seeds, fresh fruit slices

Instructions:

In a blender, combine the frozen banana slices, mixed berries, coconut milk or almond milk, and almond butter or cashew butter.

Blend until smooth and creamy, adding more liquid if needed to reach your desired consistency.

Pour the smoothie into a bowl.

Top the smoothie bowl with sliced almonds, shredded coconut, chia seeds, and fresh fruit slices for added texture and flavor.

Enjoy this delightful and nutritious Paleo Breakfast Smoothie Bowl with a spoon!

Paleo Sweet Potato and Kale Breakfast Hash

Ingredients:

2 medium sweet potatoes, peeled and diced

2 cups kale, stems removed and chopped

1 onion, diced

2 cloves garlic, minced

4 eggs

2 tablespoons coconut oil or ghee

Salt and pepper to taste

Optional: paprika or chili powder for added flavor

Instructions:

Heat coconut oil or ghee in a large skillet over medium heat.

Add diced sweet potatoes to the skillet and cook for about 8-10 minutes, stirring occasionally, until they start to soften.

Add diced onion to the skillet and cook for an additional 3-4 minutes until translucent.

Stir in minced garlic and cook for another minute until fragrant.

Add chopped kale to the skillet and cook, stirring occasionally, for 3-4 minutes until wilted and tender.

Create small wells in the hash for the eggs.

Crack one egg into each well.

Cover the skillet and cook for about 5-7 minutes or until the eggs are cooked to your desired level (for runny yolks, cook for less time).

Season with salt, pepper, and optional spices like paprika or chili powder.

Once done, remove from heat and serve this flavorful and nutritious Paleo Sweet Potato and Kale Breakfast Hash warm.

Paleo Coconut Flour Pancakes

Ingredients:

4 eggs

1/4 cup coconut milk

1/4 cup coconut flour

2 tablespoons maple syrup or honey (optional, for sweetness)

1/2 teaspoon baking powder

1/4 teaspoon vanilla extract

Pinch of salt

Coconut oil for cooking

Instructions:

In a mixing bowl, whisk together the eggs, coconut milk, maple syrup or honey (if using), and vanilla extract until well combined.

In a separate bowl, mix the coconut flour, baking powder, and a pinch of salt.

Gradually add the dry ingredients to the wet ingredients, stirring until there are no lumps and the batter is smooth. Let the batter rest for a few minutes to allow the coconut flour to absorb the liquid.

Heat a skillet or griddle over medium heat and lightly grease it with coconut oil.

Pour small amounts of the pancake batter onto the skillet to form pancakes.

Cook for about 2-3 minutes on each side until golden brown, flipping carefully.

Once cooked, remove the pancakes from the skillet and continue cooking the remaining batter.

Serve the Paleo Coconut Flour Pancakes warm with a drizzle of maple syrup, fresh fruit, or a dollop of coconut yogurt for added flavor.

Egg Muffins

Ingredients:

6 eggs

1 cup diced vegetables (bell peppers, spinach, tomatoes, onions, etc.)

1/2 cup cooked and crumbled bacon or diced ham (optional)

Salt and pepper to taste

Coconut oil or ghee for greasing the muffin tin

Instructions:

Preheat your oven to 350°F (175°C) and grease a muffin tin with coconut oil or ghee.

In a mixing bowl, whisk the eggs together until well beaten. Season with salt and pepper.

Distribute the diced vegetables and bacon or ham (if using) evenly among the muffin tin compartments.

Pour the beaten eggs over the vegetables and meat in the muffin tin, filling each compartment about three-quarters full.

Place the muffin tin in the preheated oven and bake for 20-25 minutes or until the egg muffins are set and slightly golden on top.

Once done, remove the egg muffins from the oven and let them cool for a few minutes.

Gently remove the egg muffins from the tin using a spoon or knife.

Veggie and Herb Frittata

Ingredients:

8 eggs

1 cup mixed vegetables (bell peppers, spinach, tomatoes, onions, etc.), chopped

1/4 cup fresh herbs (such as parsley, basil, or cilantro), chopped

2 tablespoons olive oil or coconut oil

Salt and pepper to taste

Instructions:

Preheat your oven to 350°F (175°C).

In a mixing bowl, crack the eggs and whisk them together until well combined.

Heat olive oil or coconut oil in an oven-safe skillet over medium heat.

Add the chopped vegetables to the skillet and sauté for about 3-4 minutes until they begin to soften.

Pour the whisked eggs over the sautéed vegetables in the skillet.

Sprinkle the fresh herbs evenly over the egg mixture.

Season with salt and pepper to taste.

Allow the frittata to cook on the stovetop for about 3-4 minutes until the edges start to set.

Transfer the skillet to the preheated oven and bake for 12-15 minutes or until the frittata is fully set in the center and slightly golden on top.

Once done, remove the skillet from the oven and let it cool for a few minutes.

Slice the frittata into wedges and serve warm.

Banana Almond Butter Chia Seed Pudding

Ingredients:

2 ripe bananas

1/4 cup almond butter

2 cups coconut milk or almond milk

1/2 cup chia seeds

1 teaspoon vanilla extract

Optional toppings: sliced bananas, chopped nuts, shredded coconut

Instructions:

In a blender, combine the ripe bananas, almond butter, coconut milk or almond milk, and vanilla extract. Blend until smooth.

Transfer the blended mixture to a bowl or container.

Add the chia seeds to the bowl and stir well to combine.

Cover the bowl or container and refrigerate the mixture for at least 4 hours or overnight, allowing the chia seeds to absorb the liquid and thicken the pudding.

Before serving, give the pudding a good stir to ensure it's evenly mixed and creamy.

Divide the chia seed pudding into serving bowls.

Top with sliced bananas, chopped nuts, shredded coconut, or any other toppings of your choice.

Paleo Breakfast Burrito Bowl

Ingredients:

4 large eggs

1 avocado, sliced

1 sweet potato, diced

1 red bell pepper, diced

1 small onion, diced

1 teaspoon paprika

1 teaspoon cumin

2 tablespoons olive oil or coconut oil

Salt and pepper to taste

Fresh cilantro for garnish (optional)

Salsa or hot sauce (optional)

Instructions:

Preheat your oven to 400°F (200°C).

Place the diced sweet potato on a baking sheet, drizzle with olive oil or melted coconut oil, and sprinkle with paprika, cumin, salt, and pepper. Toss to coat evenly.

Roast the sweet potatoes in the preheated oven for about 20-25 minutes until they are tender and slightly crispy.

In a skillet over medium heat, add a tablespoon of olive oil or coconut oil.

Sauté the diced onion and red bell pepper until they are softened and slightly caramelized, about 5-7 minutes.

Crack the eggs into the skillet with the sautéed vegetables and scramble them until they are cooked to your desired consistency.

Assemble the breakfast bowl by placing a serving of the scrambled eggs and sautéed vegetables in a bowl.

Add a portion of roasted sweet potatoes and sliced avocado on top.

Garnish with fresh cilantro and serve with salsa or hot sauce if desired.

Sausage Patties

Ingredients:

1 pound ground pork (preferably pasture-raised)

1 teaspoon dried sage

1/2 teaspoon dried thyme

1/2 teaspoon garlic powder

1/2 teaspoon onion powder

1/4 teaspoon smoked paprika

1/4 teaspoon black pepper

1/2 teaspoon salt (adjust to taste)

1-2 tablespoons coconut oil or ghee (for cooking)

Instructions:

In a mixing bowl, combine the ground pork with all the herbs and spices: dried sage, dried thyme, garlic powder, onion powder, smoked paprika, black pepper, and salt. Mix well to evenly distribute the seasonings throughout the meat.

Divide the seasoned pork mixture into equal portions and shape them into patties, about 2-3 inches in diameter.

Heat coconut oil or ghee in a skillet over medium heat.

Once the skillet is hot, add the sausage patties, making sure not to overcrowd the pan. Cook for about 3-4 minutes per side until they are browned and cooked through.

Use a spatula to flip the patties carefully to avoid breaking them.

Once cooked, transfer the sausage patties to a plate lined with a paper towel to absorb any excess oil.

Serve these flavorful Paleo Breakfast Sausage Patties alongside your favorite breakfast sides or as a protein-packed addition to your morning meal.

Apple Cinnamon Breakfast Bake

Ingredients:

4 medium apples, peeled and diced

4 eggs

1/2 cup almond flour

1/4 cup coconut flour

1/4 cup coconut oil, melted

1/4 cup maple syrup or honey

1 teaspoon cinnamon

1/2 teaspoon baking soda

1/4 teaspoon salt

Chopped nuts (optional, for topping)

Instructions:

Preheat your oven to 350°F (175°C) and grease a baking dish with coconut oil.

In a large mixing bowl, whisk the eggs until well beaten.

Add the melted coconut oil and maple syrup (or honey) to the eggs, and whisk until thoroughly combined.

Stir in the almond flour, coconut flour, cinnamon, baking soda, and salt, mixing until you have a smooth batter.

Gently fold in the diced apples into the batter.

Pour the mixture into the greased baking dish, spreading it evenly.

Optionally, sprinkle chopped nuts on top of the mixture for added texture and flavor.

Bake in the preheated oven for 35-40 minutes or until the top is golden brown and a toothpick inserted into the center comes out clean.

Once done, remove the breakfast bake from the oven and let it cool for a few minutes before slicing and serving.

Paleo Breakfast Smoothie

Ingredients:

1 ripe banana

1/2 cup mixed berries (such as strawberries, blueberries, raspberries)

1/2 cup coconut milk or almond milk

1 tablespoon almond butter or cashew butter

1 tablespoon chia seeds

1 teaspoon honey or maple syrup (optional, for added sweetness)

Ice cubes (optional)

Instructions:

Place all the ingredients in a blender.

Blend until smooth and creamy. If desired, add ice cubes for a chilled consistency.

Taste and adjust sweetness by adding honey or maple syrup, if needed.

Pour the smoothie into a glass and enjoy this nutrient-packed Paleo Breakfast Smoothie.

PALEO DIET LUNCH RECIPES

Paleo Turkey and Avocado Lettuce Wraps

Ingredients:

1 pound ground turkey

1 tablespoon olive oil

1 onion, diced

2 cloves garlic, minced

1 teaspoon ground cumin

1 teaspoon paprika

Salt and pepper to taste

1-2 avocados, sliced

Juice of 1 lime

1 head iceberg or butter lettuce, leaves separated and cleaned

Optional toppings: diced tomatoes, chopped cilantro, hot sauce

Instructions:

Heat olive oil in a skillet over medium heat. Add diced onions and sauté until translucent, then add minced garlic and cook for another minute.

Add ground turkey to the skillet and cook until browned, breaking it apart with a spatula as it cooks.

Season the turkey with ground cumin, paprika, salt, and pepper. Stir well to combine the spices evenly.

Once the turkey is cooked through, remove the skillet from heat and squeeze lime juice over the meat. Mix to incorporate the lime flavor.

Wash and dry the lettuce leaves. These will act as your wraps.

Assemble the wraps: Place a spoonful of the cooked turkey mixture onto a lettuce leaf, add a few slices of avocado on top, and sprinkle with optional toppings like diced tomatoes, cilantro, or hot sauce if desired.

Roll up the lettuce leaf to form a wrap, securing the filling inside.

Salmon and Veggie Stir-Fry?

Ingredients:

2 salmon fillets, skin removed, cut into cubes

2 tablespoons coconut oil

2 cloves garlic, minced

1-inch piece of fresh ginger, peeled and minced

1 bell pepper, sliced

1 cup broccoli florets

1 carrot, julienned or sliced

2 tablespoons coconut aminos (Paleo-friendly soy sauce alternative)

Salt and pepper to taste

Optional toppings: sesame seeds, chopped green onions

Instructions:

Heat 1 tablespoon of coconut oil in a large skillet or wok over medium-high heat.

Add minced garlic and ginger to the skillet and sauté for about a minute until fragrant.

Add the cubed salmon to the skillet and cook until browned on all sides. Remove the salmon from the skillet and set aside.

In the same skillet, add another tablespoon of coconut oil if needed. Add the sliced bell pepper, broccoli florets, and julienned carrot. Stir-fry the vegetables until they are tender-crisp.

Return the cooked salmon to the skillet with the vegetables.

Pour in the coconut aminos and toss everything together to coat evenly. Season with salt and pepper to taste.

Cook for an additional 2-3 minutes until the salmon is heated through and the flavors meld together.

Serve the salmon and vegetable stir-fry hot, garnished with sesame seeds and chopped green onions if desired.

Paleo Chicken Lettuce Wraps:

Ingredients:

1 lb ground chicken

2 tablespoons coconut oil

1 onion, finely chopped

2 cloves garlic, minced

1 red bell pepper, diced

1 cup mushrooms, chopped

2 tablespoons coconut aminos (Paleo-friendly soy sauce substitute)

1 teaspoon sesame oil

Salt and pepper to taste

Butter lettuce leaves for wrapping

Instructions:

Heat coconut oil in a skillet over medium heat.

Add chopped onions and minced garlic, sauté until fragrant.

Add ground chicken to the skillet, breaking it up with a spatula as it cooks. Cook until it's no longer pink.

Add diced bell pepper and chopped mushrooms to the skillet. Cook for a few minutes until the vegetables start to soften.

Pour in the coconut aminos and sesame oil, stirring to combine. Season with salt and pepper to taste. Cook for an additional 2-3 minutes.

Wash and dry the butter lettuce leaves, which will be used as wraps.

Spoon the chicken and vegetable mixture onto the lettuce leaves.

Serve the chicken lettuce wraps immediately.

Cauliflower Fried Rice with Shrimp?

Ingredients:

1 head cauliflower, grated or processed into rice-like texture

1 tablespoon coconut oil

1 pound shrimp, peeled and deveined

2 cloves garlic, minced

1-inch piece of ginger, grated

1 cup mixed vegetables (such as diced carrots, peas, bell peppers)

2 tablespoons coconut aminos (Paleo-friendly soy sauce substitute)

2 eggs, beaten

Salt and pepper to taste

Optional: chopped green onions for garnish

Instructions:

Heat coconut oil in a large skillet or wok over medium-high heat.

Add minced garlic and grated ginger to the skillet, sauté for about a minute until fragrant.

Add the shrimp to the skillet and cook until they turn pink and are cooked through. Remove the shrimp from the skillet and set aside.

In the same skillet, add the mixed vegetables and stir-fry until they start to soften.

Push the vegetables to the side of the skillet, and pour the beaten eggs into the empty space. Scramble the eggs until cooked, then mix them with the vegetables.

Add the cauliflower rice to the skillet and stir-fry for a few minutes until it's heated through and slightly tender.

Return the cooked shrimp to the skillet.

Pour the coconut aminos over the cauliflower rice and shrimp. Toss everything together until well combined. Season with salt and pepper to taste.

Cook for an additional 2-3 minutes, ensuring everything is heated through.

Garnish with chopped green onions if desired and serve hot.

Turkey and Sweet Potato Hash:

Ingredients:

1 pound ground turkey

2 tablespoons olive oil or coconut oil

2 medium sweet potatoes, peeled and diced into small cubes

1 onion, diced

2 cloves garlic, minced

1 teaspoon paprika

1 teaspoon dried thyme

Salt and pepper to taste

Chopped fresh parsley for garnish (optional)

Instructions:

Heat the olive oil or coconut oil in a large skillet over medium-high heat.

Add the diced sweet potatoes to the skillet and cook for about 5-7 minutes, stirring occasionally, until they start to soften.

Add the diced onion to the skillet and sauté for a few minutes until the onions become translucent.

Push the sweet potatoes and onions to the side of the skillet and add the ground turkey to the empty space. Break up the turkey with a spatula and cook until it's no longer pink.

Stir the sweet potatoes, onions, and turkey together in the skillet.

Add minced garlic, paprika, dried thyme, salt, and pepper to the mixture. Mix everything thoroughly.

Cook for an additional 5-7 minutes, or until the sweet potatoes are tender and the turkey is cooked through.

Remove the skillet from heat. Garnish with chopped fresh parsley if desired.

Serve the Paleo Turkey and Sweet Potato Hash hot.

Chicken and Vegetable Stir-Fry:

Ingredients:

1 pound chicken breasts, sliced into strips

2 tablespoons coconut oil

2 cloves garlic, minced

1-inch piece of ginger, grated

1 red bell pepper, sliced

1 yellow bell pepper, sliced

1 cup broccoli florets

1 cup snap peas, ends trimmed

2 tablespoons coconut aminos (Paleo-friendly soy sauce substitute)

Salt and pepper to taste

Optional: sesame seeds for garnish

Instructions:

Heat 1 tablespoon of coconut oil in a large skillet or wok over medium-high heat.

Add minced garlic and grated ginger to the skillet, sauté for about a minute until fragrant.

Add chicken strips to the skillet and stir-fry until they're cooked through. Remove the chicken from the skillet and set aside.

In the same skillet, add another tablespoon of coconut oil if needed. Add sliced bell peppers, broccoli florets, and snap peas. Stir-fry for a few minutes until the vegetables are tender-crisp.

Return the cooked chicken to the skillet with the vegetables.

Pour in the coconut aminos and toss everything together to coat evenly. Season with salt and pepper to taste.

Cook for an additional 2-3 minutes until everything is heated through and well combined.

Garnish with sesame seeds if desired.

Serve the Paleo Chicken and Vegetable Stir-Fry hot.

Paleo Taco Salad

Ingredients:

1 pound ground beef or turkey

1 tablespoon olive oil

1 onion, diced

2 cloves garlic, minced

1 tablespoon chili powder

1 teaspoon ground cumin

1/2 teaspoon paprika

Salt and pepper to taste

Mixed salad greens

Sliced cherry tomatoes

Sliced avocado

Sliced black olives

Chopped cilantro (optional)

Lime wedges (for garnish)

Instructions:

Heat olive oil in a skillet over medium-high heat.

Add diced onion and minced garlic to the skillet. Sauté until the onions become translucent.

Add ground beef or turkey to the skillet and cook until browned, breaking it apart with a spatula as it cooks.

Season the meat with chili powder, ground cumin, paprika, salt, and pepper. Stir well to combine the spices evenly.

Cook the meat for an additional 5-7 minutes until it's fully cooked and the flavors meld together.

Assemble the salad: Start with a bed of mixed salad greens in a bowl or plate. Top it with the cooked taco meat, sliced cherry tomatoes, avocado slices, black olives, and chopped cilantro if desired.

Squeeze lime wedges over the salad for extra flavor.

Toss everything together gently or serve as is.

Paleo-style Zucchini Noodle Stir-Fry

Ingredients:

3 medium zucchinis, spiralized or cut into noodle shapes

1 tablespoon coconut oil

2 chicken breasts, thinly sliced

2 cloves garlic, minced

1-inch piece of ginger, grated

1 red bell pepper, thinly sliced

1 cup snap peas, ends trimmed

2 tablespoons coconut aminos (Paleo-friendly soy sauce substitute)

1 tablespoon sesame oil

Salt and pepper to taste

Optional: chopped green onions or sesame seeds for garnish

Instructions:

Heat coconut oil in a large skillet or wok over medium-high heat.

Add minced garlic and grated ginger to the skillet, sauté for about a minute until fragrant.

Add sliced chicken breasts to the skillet and stir-fry until they're cooked through. Remove the chicken from the skillet and set aside.

In the same skillet, add the sliced bell pepper and snap peas. Stir-fry for a few minutes until they start to soften.

Add the zucchini noodles to the skillet. Stir-fry for 2-3 minutes until the noodles are just tender but still have a slight crunch.

Return the cooked chicken to the skillet with the vegetables and zucchini noodles.

Pour in the coconut aminos and sesame oil. Toss everything together to coat evenly. Season with salt and pepper to taste.

Cook for an additional 2-3 minutes until everything is heated through.

Garnish with chopped green onions or sesame seeds if desired.

Serve the Paleo Zucchini Noodle Stir-Fry hot.

Tuna Salad Stuffed Avocado

Ingredients:

2 cans of tuna, drained

2 ripe avocados

1/4 cup red onion, finely chopped

1/4 cup cucumber, diced

1/4 cup cherry tomatoes, halved

1 tablespoon fresh lemon juice

2 tablespoons olive oil

Salt and pepper to taste

Optional: chopped fresh parsley or cilantro for garnish

Instructions:

In a mixing bowl, combine drained tuna, chopped red onion, diced cucumber, and halved cherry tomatoes.

Drizzle olive oil and fresh lemon juice over the tuna mixture. Season with salt and pepper according to taste. Mix everything together until well combined.

Cut the avocados in half and remove the pits. Scoop out a little extra avocado flesh to create a larger space for the tuna salad.

Divide the tuna salad among the avocado halves, filling the centers generously.

Optionally, garnish with chopped fresh parsley or cilantro.

Serve the Paleo Tuna Salad Stuffed Avocado immediately.

Grilled Chicken Salad with Mango Salsa?

Ingredients:

For the Grilled Chicken:

2 boneless, skinless chicken breasts

2 tablespoons olive oil

1 teaspoon paprika

1 teaspoon garlic powder

Salt and pepper to taste

For the Mango Salsa:

1 ripe mango, peeled and diced

1/2 red onion, finely chopped

1 red bell pepper, diced

1 jalapeño, seeded and finely chopped

Juice of 1 lime

2 tablespoons chopped fresh cilantro

Salt to taste

For the Salad:

Mixed salad greens

Sliced cucumber

Sliced avocado

Instructions:

Preheat the grill to medium-high heat.

In a bowl, mix olive oil, paprika, garlic powder, salt, and pepper. Coat the chicken breasts with this mixture.

Grill the chicken breasts for about 6-8 minutes per side, or until they are cooked through and have nice grill marks. Set aside to rest for a few minutes before slicing.

For the Mango Salsa:

In a separate bowl, combine diced mango, red onion, red bell pepper, jalapeño, lime juice, cilantro, and salt. Mix well. Adjust seasoning if needed.

Assembling the Salad:

Arrange mixed salad greens, sliced cucumber, and avocado on a plate.

Slice the grilled chicken breasts and place them on top of the salad.

Spoon the mango salsa over the chicken and salad.

Optionally, drizzle with a bit of extra lime juice and sprinkle with additional cilantro.

Cauliflower Rice Bowl with Sautéed Vegetables and Shrimp

Ingredients:

1 pound shrimp, peeled and deveined

1 head cauliflower, grated or processed into rice-like texture

2 tablespoons coconut oil

1 onion, finely chopped

2 cloves garlic, minced

1 red bell pepper, sliced

1 yellow bell pepper, sliced

1 cup broccoli florets

2 tablespoons coconut aminos (Paleo-friendly soy sauce substitute)

Salt and pepper to taste

Optional: chopped cilantro for garnish

Instructions:

Heat 1 tablespoon of coconut oil in a large skillet or wok over medium-high heat.

Add minced garlic and finely chopped onion to the skillet, sauté for about a minute until fragrant.

Add shrimp to the skillet and cook until they turn pink and are cooked through. Remove the shrimp from the skillet and set aside.

In the same skillet, add another tablespoon of coconut oil if needed. Add sliced bell peppers and broccoli florets. Sauté for a few minutes until they start to soften.

Add the grated cauliflower to the skillet. Stir-fry for 5-7 minutes until the cauliflower is tender but not mushy.

Return the cooked shrimp to the skillet with the vegetables and cauliflower rice.

Pour in the coconut aminos. Toss everything together to coat evenly. Season with salt and pepper to taste.

Cook for an additional 2-3 minutes until everything is heated through.

Garnish with chopped cilantro if desired.

Serve the Paleo Cauliflower Rice Bowl with Sautéed Vegetables and Shrimp hot.

Paleo Egg Roll

Ingredients:

1 pound ground pork or turkey

1 tablespoon coconut oil

1 onion, thinly sliced

3 cloves garlic, minced

1 teaspoon fresh ginger, grated

1 head cabbage, thinly sliced

2 carrots, julienned or grated

1/4 cup coconut aminos (Paleo-friendly soy sauce substitute)

1 tablespoon rice vinegar

1 teaspoon sesame oil

Salt and pepper to taste

Optional: sliced green onions for garnish

Instructions:

Heat coconut oil in a large skillet or wok over medium-high heat.

Add ground pork or turkey to the skillet and cook until browned, breaking it apart as it cooks. Once cooked, remove from the skillet and set aside.

In the same skillet, add sliced onions and sauté until they start to soften.

Add minced garlic and grated ginger to the skillet. Sauté for another minute until fragrant.

Add sliced cabbage and julienned/grated carrots to the skillet. Stir-fry for a few minutes until the vegetables begin to wilt and soften.

Return the cooked pork or turkey to the skillet with the vegetables.

Pour in the coconut aminos, rice vinegar, and sesame oil. Mix everything together to combine. Season with salt and pepper to taste.

Cook for an additional 2-3 minutes until everything is heated through and flavors are well combined.

Garnish with sliced green onions if desired.

Serve the Paleo Egg Roll in a Bowl hot.

Paleo Butternut Squash

Ingredients:

1 medium-sized butternut squash, peeled, seeds removed, and diced

1 onion, chopped

2 cloves garlic, minced

1 carrot, peeled and chopped

2 celery stalks, chopped

4 cups chicken or vegetable broth

1 can (13.5 oz) coconut milk

2 tablespoons olive oil or coconut oil

1 teaspoon ground cinnamon

1/2 teaspoon ground nutmeg

Salt and pepper to taste

Optional: fresh parsley or chives for garnish

Instructions:

In a large pot, heat olive oil or coconut oil over medium heat.

Add chopped onion, minced garlic, chopped carrot, and chopped celery to the pot. Sauté for about 5 minutes until the vegetables start to soften.

Add diced butternut squash to the pot and sauté for an additional 5 minutes.

Pour in the chicken or vegetable broth. Bring the mixture to a boil, then reduce the heat to simmer.

Cover and simmer for about 20-25 minutes, or until the butternut squash is tender.

Using an immersion blender or regular blender, puree the soup until smooth. If using a regular blender, blend in batches and be cautious of hot liquids.

Return the pureed soup to the pot (if using a regular blender) and place it back on the stove over low heat.

Stir in the coconut milk, ground cinnamon, ground nutmeg, salt, and pepper. Simmer for another 5-10 minutes, stirring occasionally.

Adjust seasoning if needed.

Serve the Paleo Butternut Squash Soup hot, garnished with fresh parsley or chives if desired.

Chicken and Vegetable Skewers with Chimichurri Sauce

Ingredients:

For the Chicken and Vegetable Skewers:

1 pound boneless, skinless chicken breasts, cut into cubes

1 zucchini, sliced

1 red bell pepper, cut into chunks

1 yellow bell pepper, cut into chunks

1 red onion, cut into chunks

Wooden or metal skewers (if using wooden skewers, soak them in water for 30 minutes before using)

For the Marinade:

1/4 cup olive oil

2 tablespoons fresh lemon juice

2 cloves garlic, minced

1 teaspoon dried oregano

1 teaspoon paprika

Salt and pepper to taste

For the Chimichurri Sauce:

1 cup fresh parsley leaves, finely chopped

1/4 cup fresh cilantro leaves, finely chopped

2 cloves garlic, minced

1 shallot, finely chopped

1/4 cup red wine vinegar

1/2 cup olive oil

1/2 teaspoon red pepper flakes (adjust to taste)

Salt and pepper to taste

Instructions:

In a bowl, mix together the ingredients for the marinade: olive oil, lemon juice, minced garlic, dried oregano, paprika, salt, and pepper. Add the cubed chicken to the marinade, ensuring it's coated well. Allow it to marinate in the refrigerator for at least 30 minutes.

Preheat the grill or grill pan to medium-high heat.

Thread the marinated chicken cubes, zucchini slices, red and yellow bell pepper chunks, and red onion chunks onto skewers, alternating between the ingredients.

Grill the skewers for about 8-10 minutes, turning occasionally, until the chicken is cooked through and the vegetables are tender and lightly charred.

While the skewers are cooking, prepare the chimichurri sauce. In a bowl, combine the finely chopped parsley, cilantro, minced garlic, chopped shallot, red wine vinegar, olive oil, red pepper flakes, salt, and pepper. Mix well to combine.

Once the skewers are cooked, remove them from the grill and serve hot with the chimichurri sauce drizzled over the top or served on the side.

Turkey and Veggie Stir-Fry

Ingredients:

1 pound ground turkey

2 tablespoons coconut oil

1 onion, thinly sliced

2 cloves garlic, minced

1 red bell pepper, sliced

1 yellow bell pepper, sliced

1 cup snow peas, trimmed

1 cup sliced mushrooms

2 tablespoons coconut aminos (Paleo-friendly soy sauce substitute)

Salt and pepper to taste

Optional: chopped fresh cilantro for garnish

Instructions:

Heat coconut oil in a large skillet or wok over medium-high heat.

Add thinly sliced onion and minced garlic to the skillet. Sauté for a few minutes until the onions become translucent.

Add ground turkey to the skillet and cook until it's browned and cooked through. Break up the turkey with a spatula as it cooks.

Add sliced red and yellow bell peppers, snow peas, and sliced mushrooms to the skillet. Stir-fry for a few minutes until the vegetables start to soften but remain crisp.

Pour in the coconut aminos (or Paleo-friendly soy sauce substitute) over the turkey and vegetables. Toss everything together to coat evenly.

Season with salt and pepper to taste. Adjust seasoning if needed.

Cook for an additional 2-3 minutes until everything is heated through and flavors are well combined.

Garnish with chopped fresh cilantro if desired.

Serve the Paleo Turkey and Veggie Stir-Fry hot.

PALEO DIET DINNER RECIPES DINNER

Baked Lemon Garlic Salmon with Roasted Vegetables

Ingredients:

4 salmon fillets

2 tablespoons olive oil

4 cloves garlic, minced

Zest of 1 lemon

Juice of 1 lemon

2 tablespoons fresh parsley, chopped

Salt and pepper to taste

For the roasted vegetables:

2 cups broccoli florets

2 cups cauliflower florets

1 red bell pepper, sliced

1 yellow bell pepper, sliced

1 red onion, sliced

3 tablespoons olive oil

1 teaspoon dried thyme

1 teaspoon dried oregano

Salt and pepper to taste

Instructions:

Preheat your oven to 400°F (200°C).

In a small bowl, mix together olive oil, minced garlic, lemon zest, lemon juice, chopped parsley, salt, and pepper.

Place the salmon fillets on a baking sheet lined with parchment paper. Brush the lemon garlic mixture evenly over the salmon fillets.

In a separate large bowl, combine the broccoli, cauliflower, bell peppers, and onion. Drizzle with olive oil, sprinkle with dried thyme, oregano, salt, and pepper. Toss until the vegetables are evenly coated.

Spread the seasoned vegetables onto another baking sheet lined with parchment paper.

Place both the salmon and the vegetables in the preheated oven. Bake for about 12-15 minutes, or until the salmon is cooked through and flakes easily with a fork, and the vegetables are tender and slightly browned.

Once done, remove the salmon and vegetables from the oven.

Plate the baked lemon garlic salmon alongside the roasted vegetables.

Zucchini Noodles with Pesto and Grilled Shrimp

Ingredients:

1 pound large shrimp, peeled and deveined

4 medium zucchinis

2 tablespoons olive oil

Salt and pepper to taste

For the pesto:

2 cups fresh basil leaves, packed

1/3 cup pine nuts (or walnuts)

2 cloves garlic, minced

1/2 cup olive oil

1/2 cup grated Paleo-friendly cheese (such as nutritional yeast for a dairy-free option)

Salt and pepper to taste

Instructions:

Preheat a grill or grill pan over medium-high heat.

In a food processor, combine the basil leaves, pine nuts (or walnuts), minced garlic, olive oil, grated cheese, salt, and pepper. Blend until the mixture forms a smooth paste. Taste and adjust seasoning if needed. Set the pesto aside.

Using a spiralizer or vegetable peeler, create zucchini noodles (zoodles) from the zucchinis.

Toss the zucchini noodles with 2 tablespoons of olive oil, salt, and pepper.

Thread the shrimp onto skewers and brush them with a little olive oil. Season with salt and pepper.

Grill the shrimp skewers for about 2-3 minutes per side until they are cooked through and have a nice char.

While the shrimp is grilling, heat a large skillet over medium heat. Add the zucchini noodles and cook for 2-3 minutes, stirring occasionally until they are just tender.

Remove the skillet from heat and toss the zucchini noodles with the prepared pesto until they are evenly coated.

Once the shrimp is done, remove them from the grill.

Serve the zucchini noodles topped with the grilled shrimp skewers.

Stuffed Bell Peppers

Ingredients:

4 large bell peppers (any color)

1 pound ground beef (or turkey)

1 small onion, finely chopped

2 cloves garlic, minced

1 cup cauliflower rice

1 can (14 oz) diced tomatoes, drained

1 teaspoon dried oregano

1 teaspoon dried basil

Salt and pepper to taste

1 cup Paleo-friendly marinara sauce

1/2 cup grated Paleo-friendly cheese (optional, for topping)

Instructions:

Preheat your oven to 375°F (190°C).

Cut the tops off the bell peppers and remove the seeds and membranes. Rinse the peppers inside and out. Place them in a baking dish, standing upright.

In a skillet over medium heat, cook the ground beef (or turkey) until browned. Drain excess fat if needed.

Add the chopped onion and minced garlic to the skillet with the meat and cook for a few minutes until the onions are translucent.

Stir in the cauliflower rice, drained diced tomatoes, dried oregano, dried basil, salt, and pepper. Cook for an additional 5 minutes until the cauliflower rice is tender and the flavors are well combined.

Spoon the mixture into the hollowed-out bell peppers, pressing gently to fill them evenly.

Pour the marinara sauce over the stuffed peppers.

Cover the baking dish with foil and bake for about 35-40 minutes, or until the peppers are tender.

If using grated cheese, remove the foil, sprinkle the cheese over the stuffed peppers, and bake for an additional 5 minutes, or until the cheese is melted and bubbly.

Remove from the oven and let the stuffed peppers cool for a few minutes before serving.

Paleo Beef Stir-Fry

Ingredients:

1 pound beef steak (flank, sirloin, or any lean cut), thinly sliced

2 tablespoons coconut aminos (Paleo-friendly soy sauce alternative)

2 cloves garlic, minced

1-inch piece of fresh ginger, grated

2 tablespoons coconut oil or avocado oil

1 onion, sliced

2 bell peppers (any color), sliced

2 cups broccoli florets

Salt and pepper to taste

Sesame seeds for garnish (optional)

Sliced green onions for garnish (optional)

Instructions:

In a bowl, marinate the sliced beef with coconut aminos, minced garlic, and grated ginger. Let it marinate for about 15-20 minutes.

Heat a large skillet or wok over medium-high heat. Add 1 tablespoon of coconut oil.

Once the skillet is hot, add the marinated beef slices (reserving the marinade) and stir-fry for about 2-3 minutes or until the beef is browned. Remove the beef from the skillet and set it aside.

In the same skillet, add another tablespoon of coconut oil. Add the sliced onion, bell peppers, and broccoli florets. Stir-fry for about 4-5 minutes until the vegetables are tender-crisp.

Return the cooked beef to the skillet with the vegetables.

Pour the reserved marinade over the beef and vegetables. Stir well to combine and heat through for another 1-2 minutes.

Season with salt and pepper to taste.

Garnish the Paleo beef stir-fry with sesame seeds and sliced green onions if desired.

Paleo Chicken and Vegetable Curry

Ingredients:

1.5 lbs boneless, skinless chicken thighs, cut into bite-sized pieces

2 tablespoons coconut oil

1 onion, finely chopped

3 cloves garlic, minced

1 tablespoon fresh ginger, grated

2 tablespoons curry powder

1 can (14 oz) coconut milk

1 cup chicken broth

2 cups broccoli florets

2 carrots, sliced

1 red bell pepper, sliced

Salt and pepper to taste

Fresh cilantro for garnish (optional)

Cauliflower rice or steamed vegetables (optional, for serving)

Instructions:

In a large skillet or pan, heat coconut oil over medium heat. Add the chopped onion and cook until softened, about 3-4 minutes.

Add the minced garlic and grated ginger to the skillet, stirring constantly for about a minute until fragrant.

Add the chicken pieces to the skillet and cook until they are browned on all sides, about 5-6 minutes.

Sprinkle the curry powder over the chicken and vegetables, stirring well to coat everything evenly.

Pour in the coconut milk and chicken broth. Bring the mixture to a gentle simmer.

Add the broccoli florets, sliced carrots, and red bell pepper to the skillet. Stir to combine.

Cover the skillet and let the curry simmer for about 15-20 minutes, or until the chicken is cooked through and the vegetables are tender.

Season with salt and pepper to taste.

Optionally, serve the Paleo chicken and vegetable curry over cauliflower rice or alongside steamed vegetables.

Garnish with fresh cilantro for added flavor (if desired).

Paleo Turkey Sweet Potato Skillet

Ingredients:

1 pound ground turkey

2 tablespoons olive oil

2 large sweet potatoes, peeled and diced

1 bell pepper, diced

1 onion, diced

2 cloves garlic, minced

1 teaspoon paprika

1 teaspoon dried oregano

1 teaspoon dried thyme

Salt and pepper to taste

Fresh parsley or cilantro for garnish (optional)

Instructions:

Heat olive oil in a large skillet over medium heat.

Add the ground turkey to the skillet and cook, breaking it apart with a spoon, until it's no longer pink.

Once the turkey is cooked, remove it from the skillet and set it aside.

In the same skillet, add a bit more olive oil if needed. Add the diced sweet potatoes and sauté for about 8-10 minutes, or until they start to soften.

Add the diced bell pepper, onion, and minced garlic to the skillet with the sweet potatoes. Cook for an additional 5-6 minutes, stirring occasionally, until the vegetables are tender.

Return the cooked turkey to the skillet with the vegetables.

Sprinkle paprika, dried oregano, dried thyme, salt, and pepper over the mixture. Stir everything together until well combined.

Cover the skillet and let it cook for another 5-7 minutes, or until the flavors meld together, and the sweet potatoes are fully cooked.

Taste and adjust seasoning if needed.

Garnish with fresh parsley or cilantro before serving (if desired).

Grilled Lemon Herb Pork Chops

Ingredients:

4 pork chops (bone-in or boneless)

Zest of 1 lemon

Juice of 1 lemon

2 cloves garlic, minced

2 tablespoons fresh rosemary, chopped

2 tablespoons fresh thyme, chopped

2 tablespoons olive oil

Salt and pepper to taste

Instructions:

Preheat your grill to medium-high heat.

In a small bowl, combine the lemon zest, lemon juice, minced garlic, chopped rosemary, chopped thyme, olive oil, salt, and pepper to create a marinade.

Pat dry the pork chops with paper towels. Season both sides of the pork chops with additional salt and pepper if desired.

Place the pork chops in a shallow dish or a resealable plastic bag. Pour the marinade over the pork chops, ensuring they are evenly coated. Allow them to marinate in the refrigerator for at least 30 minutes, allowing the flavors to meld.

Once marinated, remove the pork chops from the marinade and discard the excess marinade.

Grill the pork chops for about 4-5 minutes on each side, depending on the thickness of the chops, or until they reach an internal temperature of 145°F (63°C) for medium-rare or up to 160°F (71°C) for medium, using a meat thermometer.

Once grilled, remove the pork chops from the grill and let them rest for a few minutes before serving.

Serve the grilled lemon herb pork chops with your choice of sides, such as roasted vegetables, a salad, or cauliflower rice.

Paleo Beef and Vegetable Stir-Fry

Ingredients:

1 pound beef sirloin or flank steak, thinly sliced

2 tablespoons coconut aminos (Paleo-friendly soy sauce substitute)

2 tablespoons olive oil or coconut oil

3 cloves garlic, minced

1-inch piece of fresh ginger, grated

1 onion, sliced

2 bell peppers (any color), sliced

2 cups broccoli florets

1 cup sliced carrots

Salt and pepper to taste

Sesame seeds for garnish (optional)

Sliced green onions for garnish (optional)

Instructions:

In a bowl, combine the thinly sliced beef with coconut aminos, minced garlic, and grated ginger. Allow it to marinate for about 15-20 minutes.

Heat a tablespoon of olive oil or coconut oil in a large skillet or wok over medium-high heat.

Add the marinated beef slices to the skillet and stir-fry for about 3-4 minutes until the beef is browned. Remove the beef from the skillet and set it aside.

In the same skillet, add another tablespoon of oil. Add the sliced onion, bell peppers, broccoli florets, and sliced carrots. Stir-fry for about 5-6 minutes until the vegetables are tender-crisp.

Return the cooked beef to the skillet with the vegetables and stir to combine.

Season the stir-fry with salt and pepper to taste.

Once everything is heated through, remove the skillet from heat.

Optionally, garnish the Paleo beef and vegetable stir-fry with sesame seeds and sliced green onions for added flavor and presentation.

Paleo Lemon Garlic Roasted Chicken Thighs

Ingredients:

6-8 chicken thighs, bone-in and skin-on

Zest of 1 lemon

Juice of 1 lemon

4 cloves garlic, minced

2 tablespoons fresh rosemary, chopped

2 tablespoons fresh thyme, chopped

3 tablespoons olive oil

Salt and pepper to taste

Instructions:

Preheat your oven to 400°F (200°C).

In a small bowl, mix together the lemon zest, lemon juice, minced garlic, chopped rosemary, chopped thyme, olive oil, salt, and pepper to create a marinade.

Pat dry the chicken thighs with paper towels. Season both sides of the chicken thighs with additional salt and pepper if desired.

Place the chicken thighs in a baking dish or a rimmed baking sheet.

Pour the prepared marinade over the chicken thighs, making sure they are coated evenly. Use your hands to rub the marinade into the chicken.

Let the chicken thighs marinate for at least 15-20 minutes, allowing the flavors to infuse.

Place the baking dish in the preheated oven and roast for about 35-40 minutes or until the chicken thighs are golden brown and cooked through. The internal temperature should reach 165°F (75°C).

Once done, remove the chicken thighs from the oven and let them rest for a few minutes before serving.

Serve the Paleo lemon garlic roasted chicken thighs with your choice of sides, such as roasted vegetables, salad, or cauliflower mash.

Paleo Baked Salmon with Roasted Vegetables

Ingredients:

4 salmon fillets

2 tablespoons olive oil

2 cloves garlic, minced

Zest of 1 lemon

1 teaspoon paprika

1 teaspoon dried oregano

Salt and pepper to taste

For the roasted vegetables:

2 cups cherry tomatoes

2 cups asparagus spears, trimmed

1 red onion, cut into wedges

2 tablespoons balsamic vinegar

2 tablespoons olive oil

1 teaspoon dried thyme

Salt and pepper to taste

Instructions:

Preheat your oven to 400°F (200°C).

In a small bowl, mix together olive oil, minced garlic, lemon zest, paprika, dried oregano, salt, and pepper.

Place the salmon fillets on a baking sheet lined with parchment paper. Brush the olive oil mixture evenly over the salmon fillets.

In a separate bowl, combine cherry tomatoes, asparagus spears, and red onion wedges. Drizzle with balsamic vinegar, olive oil, dried thyme, salt, and pepper. Toss until the vegetables are coated.

Spread the seasoned vegetables onto another baking sheet lined with parchment paper.

Place both the salmon and the vegetables in the preheated oven. Bake for about 12-15 minutes, or until the salmon is cooked through and flakes easily with a fork, and the vegetables are tender and slightly caramelized.

Once done, remove the salmon and vegetables from the oven.

Serve the baked salmon alongside the roasted vegetables for a delightful and nutritious Paleo dinner!

Paleo Cauliflower Fried Rice with Shrimp

Ingredients:

1 pound large shrimp, peeled and deveined

1 head cauliflower, grated or processed into rice-like texture

2 tablespoons coconut oil or olive oil

3 cloves garlic, minced

1 small onion, finely chopped

2 carrots, diced

1 cup frozen peas

2 eggs, beaten

3 tablespoons coconut aminos (Paleo-friendly soy sauce substitute)

1 teaspoon sesame oil

Salt and pepper to taste

Chopped green onions for garnish (optional)

Instructions:

Heat 1 tablespoon of coconut oil or olive oil in a large skillet or wok over medium-high heat.

Add the shrimp to the skillet and cook for 2-3 minutes per side until they turn pink and opaque. Remove the shrimp from the skillet and set aside.

In the same skillet, add the remaining tablespoon of oil. Sauté the minced garlic and chopped onion for about 2 minutes until they soften.

Add the diced carrots and cook for an additional 3-4 minutes until they start to soften.

Push the vegetables to one side of the skillet and pour the beaten eggs onto the other side. Scramble the eggs until they're cooked through, then mix them with the vegetables.

Add the grated cauliflower to the skillet along with frozen peas. Stir well to combine all the ingredients.

Pour the coconut aminos and sesame oil over the cauliflower mixture. Stir and cook for 4-5 minutes, allowing the cauliflower to cook through and absorb the flavors.

Finally, add the cooked shrimp back into the skillet. Season with salt and pepper to taste. Stir everything together and cook for an additional 2-3 minutes until the shrimp is heated through.

Garnish with chopped green onions if desired before serving.

Spaghetti Squash with Bolognese Sauce

Ingredients:

1 large spaghetti squash

1 pound ground beef

1 can (14 oz) crushed tomatoes

1 onion, diced

2 cloves garlic, minced

1 carrot, grated

1 celery stalk, diced

2 tablespoons tomato paste

2 tablespoons olive oil

1 teaspoon dried basil

1 teaspoon dried oregano

Salt and pepper to taste

Fresh basil leaves for garnish (optional)

Instructions:

Preheat your oven to 375°F (190°C).

Cut the spaghetti squash in half lengthwise and scoop out the seeds. Place the halves on a baking sheet, cut sides down. Bake for about 30-40 minutes, or until the squash is tender and easily pierced with a fork.

While the squash is baking, prepare the Bolognese sauce. Heat olive oil in a large skillet over medium heat.

Add the diced onion, minced garlic, grated carrot, and diced celery to the skillet. Sauté for about 5 minutes until the vegetables are softened.

Add the ground beef to the skillet and cook until browned, breaking it apart with a spoon as it cooks.

Stir in the crushed tomatoes, tomato paste, dried basil, dried oregano, salt, and pepper. Reduce the heat to low and simmer for 15-20 minutes, stirring occasionally, to let the flavors meld together.

Once the spaghetti squash is done baking, use a fork to scrape the flesh of the squash into "spaghetti" strands.

Serve the spaghetti squash topped with the Bolognese sauce.

Garnish with fresh basil leaves if desired.

Thai-Inspired Chicken Lettuce Wraps

Ingredients:

1 pound ground chicken (or turkey)

1 tablespoon coconut oil or olive oil

2 cloves garlic, minced

1 red bell pepper, diced

1 carrot, grated

1/2 cup water chestnuts, chopped (optional)

2 green onions, thinly sliced

2 tablespoons coconut aminos (Paleo-friendly soy sauce substitute)

1 tablespoon fish sauce

1 tablespoon lime juice

1 teaspoon fresh ginger, grated

Salt and pepper to taste

Butter or iceberg lettuce leaves (for wrapping)

Fresh cilantro and lime wedges for garnish (optional)

Instructions:

Heat coconut oil or olive oil in a skillet over medium heat.

Add the minced garlic and sauté for about 30 seconds until fragrant.

Add the ground chicken to the skillet and cook, breaking it apart with a spoon, until it's no longer pink.

Stir in the diced bell pepper, grated carrot, and water chestnuts (if using). Cook for another 3-4 minutes until the vegetables start to soften.

In a small bowl, mix together the coconut aminos, fish sauce, lime juice, grated ginger, salt, and pepper.

Pour the sauce mixture over the chicken and vegetable mixture in the skillet. Stir well to combine and let it simmer for 2-3 minutes.

Add the sliced green onions to the skillet, stirring to incorporate.

Wash and pat dry the lettuce leaves, then spoon the chicken mixture onto the leaves.

Garnish with fresh cilantro and serve with lime wedges for squeezing over the wraps.

Garlic Herb Roasted Pork Tenderloin

Ingredients:

1 ½ - 2 pounds pork tenderloin

4 cloves garlic, minced

2 tablespoons fresh rosemary, chopped

2 tablespoons fresh thyme, chopped

2 tablespoons olive oil

Salt and pepper to taste

Instructions:

Preheat your oven to 400°F (200°C).

In a small bowl, combine the minced garlic, chopped rosemary, chopped thyme, olive oil, salt, and pepper to create a paste.

Pat dry the pork tenderloin with paper towels. Season the pork with additional salt and pepper if desired.

Rub the garlic-herb paste all over the pork tenderloin, ensuring it's evenly coated.

Place the pork tenderloin on a baking sheet lined with parchment paper or in a roasting pan.

Roast in the preheated oven for about 20-25 minutes or until the internal temperature reaches 145°F (63°C) using a meat thermometer.

Once done, remove the pork tenderloin from the oven and let it rest for a few minutes before slicing.

Slice the roasted pork tenderloin and serve with your choice of sides, such as roasted vegetables, steamed greens, or a fresh salad.

Paleo Beef and Broccoli Stir-Fry

Ingredients:

1 ½ pounds beef sirloin or flank steak, thinly sliced

3 tablespoons coconut aminos (Paleo-friendly soy sauce substitute)

3 tablespoons olive oil or avocado oil, divided

3 cloves garlic, minced

1 teaspoon fresh ginger, grated

1 head broccoli, cut into florets

1 red bell pepper, sliced

1 onion, sliced

Salt and pepper to taste

Sesame seeds for garnish (optional)

Sliced green onions for garnish (optional)

Instructions:

In a bowl, marinate the thinly sliced beef with coconut aminos, 1 tablespoon of olive oil, minced garlic, and grated ginger. Allow it to marinate for about 15-20 minutes.

Heat 1 tablespoon of olive oil in a large skillet or wok over medium-high heat.

Add the marinated beef to the skillet and stir-fry for about 2-3 minutes until it's browned. Remove the beef from the skillet and set it aside.

In the same skillet, add another tablespoon of oil. Add the sliced onion, red bell pepper, and broccoli florets. Stir-fry for about 4-5 minutes until the vegetables are tender-crisp.

Return the cooked beef to the skillet with the vegetables and stir to combine.

Season with salt and pepper to taste.

Cook for an additional 1-2 minutes until everything is heated through.

Optionally, garnish the Paleo beef and broccoli stir-fry with sesame seeds and sliced green onions before serving.

PALEO DIET DESSERT RECIPES

DESSERTS

Paleo Chocolate Avocado Pudding

Ingredients:

2 ripe avocados

1/4 cup unsweetened cocoa powder

1/4 cup coconut milk (full-fat, canned)

1/4 cup maple syrup or honey (adjust to taste)

1 teaspoon vanilla extract

Pinch of salt

Optional toppings: fresh berries, shredded coconut, chopped nuts

Instructions:

Cut the avocados in half, remove the pit, and scoop the flesh into a food processor or blender.

Add the cocoa powder, coconut milk, maple syrup or honey, vanilla extract, and a pinch of salt to the blender or food processor.

Blend all the ingredients until smooth and creamy, scraping down the sides as needed to ensure everything is well combined.

Taste the mixture and adjust the sweetness if needed by adding more maple syrup or honey.

Transfer the pudding to serving bowls or glasses and refrigerate for at least 30 minutes to chill and set.

Before serving, optionally garnish the chocolate avocado pudding with fresh berries, shredded coconut, or chopped nuts for added texture and flavor.

Banana Almond Butter Blondies

Ingredients:

2 ripe bananas, mashed

1/2 cup almond butter (or any nut or seed butter)

1/4 cup coconut flour

1/4 cup almond flour

1/4 cup maple syrup or honey

1 teaspoon vanilla extract

1/2 teaspoon baking soda

Pinch of salt

Optional add-ins: dark chocolate chips, chopped nuts

Instructions:

Preheat your oven to 350°F (175°C). Grease or line an 8x8-inch baking dish with parchment paper.

In a mixing bowl, combine the mashed bananas, almond butter, maple syrup or honey, and vanilla extract. Mix until well combined.

Add the coconut flour, almond flour, baking soda, and a pinch of salt to the wet ingredients. Mix until a smooth batter forms.

If using, fold in dark chocolate chips or chopped nuts into the batter.

Pour the batter into the prepared baking dish and spread it out evenly.

Bake in the preheated oven for 20-25 minutes, or until the blondies are set and lightly golden on top.

Remove from the oven and allow the blondies to cool in the baking dish for a few minutes before transferring them to a wire rack to cool completely.

Once cooled, slice the blondies into squares and serve.

Paleo Berry Coconut Popsicles

Ingredients:

1 cup mixed berries (such as strawberries, blueberries, raspberries)

1 can (13.5 oz) full-fat coconut milk

2-3 tablespoons honey or maple syrup (adjust to taste)

1 teaspoon vanilla extract

Instructions:

In a blender, combine the mixed berries, coconut milk, honey or maple syrup, and vanilla extract. Blend until smooth.

Pour the berry and coconut milk mixture into popsicle molds, leaving a little space at the top for expansion.

Insert popsicle sticks into the molds.

Place the popsicle molds in the freezer and let them freeze for at least 4-6 hours or until completely solid.

Once frozen, run the molds under warm water for a few seconds to help release the popsicles.

Enjoy these refreshing and naturally sweet Paleo berry coconut popsicles as a guilt-free dessert or a refreshing snack on a warm day!

Paleo Chocolate Coconut Truffles

Ingredients:

1 cup unsweetened shredded coconut

1/3 cup coconut oil, melted

1/4 cup cocoa powder or cacao powder

2-3 tablespoons honey or maple syrup (adjust to taste)

1 teaspoon vanilla extract

Pinch of salt

Optional Coating:

Additional shredded coconut

Crushed nuts (such as almonds or pecans)

Cocoa powder or cacao powder

Instructions:

In a food processor or blender, pulse together the shredded coconut, melted coconut oil, cocoa powder, honey or maple syrup, vanilla extract, and a pinch of salt. Blend until the mixture forms a thick, sticky dough-like consistency.

Scoop out small portions of the mixture and roll them into balls about 1 inch in diameter. Place the balls on a parchment-lined baking sheet.

If desired, roll the truffles in additional shredded coconut, crushed nuts, or cocoa powder for coating.

Once all the truffles are formed and coated, place the baking sheet in the refrigerator for at least 30 minutes to allow the truffles to firm up.

After chilling, the truffles are ready to be served and enjoyed as a delightful Paleo-friendly sweet treat!

Paleo Mixed Berry Crumble

Ingredients:

For the Filling:

4 cups mixed berries (such as raspberries, blueberries, blackberries)

2 tablespoons arrowroot powder or tapioca flour

2 tablespoons honey or maple syrup

1 tablespoon lemon juice

Zest of 1 lemon

1 teaspoon vanilla extract

For the Crumble Topping:

1 cup almond flour

1/2 cup shredded unsweetened coconut

1/4 cup chopped nuts (walnuts, almonds, pecans)

2 tablespoons coconut oil, melted

2 tablespoons honey or maple syrup

1 teaspoon ground cinnamon

Pinch of salt

Instructions:

Preheat your oven to 350°F (175°C).

In a mixing bowl, combine the mixed berries, arrowroot powder (or tapioca flour), honey or maple syrup, lemon juice, lemon zest, and vanilla extract. Toss until the berries are evenly coated.

Transfer the berry mixture into a baking dish, spreading it out evenly.

In another bowl, mix together the almond flour, shredded coconut, chopped nuts, melted coconut oil, honey or maple syrup, ground cinnamon, and a pinch of salt. Use your fingers to create a crumbly texture.

Spread the crumble topping evenly over the berry mixture in the baking dish.

Place the dish in the preheated oven and bake for about 25-30 minutes, or until the topping is golden brown and the berry filling is bubbling.

Remove from the oven and let it cool for a few minutes before serving.

Coconut Flour Chocolate Chip Cookies

Ingredients:

1/2 cup coconut flour

1/2 cup coconut oil, melted

1/3 cup honey or maple syrup

2 eggs

1 teaspoon vanilla extract

1/4 teaspoon baking soda

Pinch of salt

1/2 cup dairy-free dark chocolate chips

Instructions:

Preheat your oven to 350°F (175°C). Line a baking sheet with parchment paper.

In a mixing bowl, combine the melted coconut oil, honey or maple syrup, eggs, and vanilla extract. Whisk until well combined.

In a separate bowl, mix together the coconut flour, baking soda, and a pinch of salt.

Gradually add the dry ingredients to the wet ingredients, stirring until a dough forms.

Fold in the dark chocolate chips into the cookie dough.

Using a spoon or cookie scoop, portion the dough and form it into balls. Place them on the prepared baking sheet, leaving some space between each cookie.

Gently flatten each cookie with the back of a spoon or your fingers.

Bake in the preheated oven for about 10-12 minutes, or until the edges are golden brown.

Once done, remove the cookies from the oven and let them cool on the baking sheet for a few minutes before transferring them to a wire rack to cool completely.

Lemon Blueberry Mug Cake

Ingredients:

3 tablespoons almond flour

1 tablespoon coconut flour

1 tablespoon coconut oil, melted

1 tablespoon honey or maple syrup

1 egg

Zest of 1 lemon

Juice of 1/2 lemon

1/4 teaspoon baking powder

1/4 cup fresh blueberries

Instructions:

In a microwave-safe mug, combine the almond
flour, coconut flour, melted coconut oil, honey

or maple syrup, egg, lemon zest, lemon juice, and baking powder. Mix until well combined.

Gently fold in the fresh blueberries into the mug cake batter.

Microwave the mug cake on high for 1.5 to 2 minutes, depending on your microwave's power. The cake should rise and set in the center.

Carefully remove the mug from the microwave (it will be hot), and allow the cake to cool for a minute.

Optionally, garnish with additional blueberries or a drizzle of honey on top.

Pumpkin Pie Bars

Ingredients:

For the Crust:

1 1/2 cups almond flour

1/4 cup coconut flour

1/4 cup coconut oil, melted

2 tablespoons maple syrup or honey

Pinch of salt

For the Pumpkin Filling:

1 can (15 oz) pumpkin puree

1/3 cup full-fat coconut milk

1/3 cup maple syrup or honey

2 eggs

1 teaspoon vanilla extract

1 teaspoon ground cinnamon

1/2 teaspoon ground ginger

1/4 teaspoon ground nutmeg

Pinch of cloves

Pinch of salt

Instructions:

Preheat your oven to 350°F (175°C). Line an 8x8-inch baking dish with parchment paper, leaving some overhang for easy removal.

In a bowl, combine almond flour, coconut flour, melted coconut oil, maple syrup or honey, and a pinch of salt. Mix until it forms a dough-like consistency.

Press the dough evenly into the bottom of the prepared baking dish to form the crust.

Bake the crust in the preheated oven for 10-12 minutes, or until lightly golden. Remove from the oven and let it cool slightly.

In another bowl, whisk together pumpkin puree, coconut milk, maple syrup or honey, eggs, vanilla extract, cinnamon, ginger, nutmeg, cloves, and a pinch of salt until well combined.

Pour the pumpkin filling over the partially baked crust, spreading it out evenly.

Return the baking dish to the oven and bake for 30-35 minutes, or until the filling is set and the edges are slightly golden.

Once done, remove from the oven and let it cool completely in the baking dish.

Once cooled, lift the bars using the parchment paper overhang, transfer to a cutting board, and slice into bars.

Chocolate Avocado Mousse

Ingredients:

2 ripe avocados

1/4 cup unsweetened cocoa powder or cacao powder

1/4 cup coconut milk (full-fat, canned)

3-4 tablespoons maple syrup or honey (adjust to taste)

1 teaspoon vanilla extract

Pinch of salt

Optional toppings: sliced berries, shredded coconut, chopped nuts

Instructions:

Cut the avocados in half, remove the pits, and scoop the flesh into a food processor or blender.

Add the cocoa powder, coconut milk, maple syrup or honey, vanilla extract, and a pinch of salt to the blender or food processor.

Blend all the ingredients until smooth and creamy, scraping down the sides as needed to ensure everything is well combined.

Taste the mixture and adjust the sweetness if needed by adding more maple syrup or honey.

Transfer the chocolate avocado mousse into serving bowls or glasses.

Optionally, top the mousse with sliced berries, shredded coconut, or chopped nuts for added texture and flavor.

Refrigerate the mousse for at least 30 minutes before serving to chill and set slightly.

Apple Cinnamon Baked Apples

Ingredients:

4 medium-sized apples (such as Granny Smith or Honeycrisp)

1/4 cup almond flour

1/4 cup chopped pecans or walnuts

2 tablespoons coconut oil, melted

2 tablespoons honey or maple syrup

1 teaspoon ground cinnamon

1/4 teaspoon ground nutmeg

Pinch of salt

Optional: Raisins or dried cranberries for extra sweetness

Instructions:

Preheat your oven to 375°F (190°C). Grease a baking dish that can hold the apples snugly.

Wash the apples and core them, leaving the bottom intact to create a well for the filling. You can use an apple corer or a small knife to carefully remove the cores and seeds.

In a bowl, combine the almond flour, chopped nuts, melted coconut oil, honey or maple syrup, ground cinnamon, ground nutmeg, and a pinch of salt. Mix until it forms a crumbly mixture.

If desired, mix in a handful of raisins or dried cranberries into the filling mixture.

Stuff each cored apple with the filling mixture, pressing it down gently.

Place the stuffed apples in the greased baking dish.

Bake in the preheated oven for about 25-30 minutes, or until the apples are tender and the filling is golden brown.

Remove from the oven and let the baked apples cool slightly before serving.

Berry Chia Seed Pudding

Ingredients:

1 cup mixed berries (strawberries, blueberries, raspberries)

1 1/2 cups coconut milk (full-fat, canned)

1/4 cup chia seeds

2-3 tablespoons honey or maple syrup (adjust to taste)

1 teaspoon vanilla extract

Optional toppings: Fresh berries, shredded coconut, sliced almonds

Instructions:

In a blender or food processor, blend the mixed berries until they form a smooth puree.

In a mixing bowl, combine the berry puree, coconut milk, chia seeds, honey or maple syrup, and vanilla extract. Mix well until all ingredients are thoroughly combined.

Cover the bowl and refrigerate the mixture for at least 4 hours or overnight, allowing the chia seeds to absorb the liquid and create a pudding-like consistency. Stir occasionally during this time to ensure the chia seeds are evenly distributed.

Once the chia seed pudding has thickened to your desired consistency, give it a final stir.

Serve the berry chia seed pudding in individual bowls or glasses.

Optionally, top the pudding with fresh berries, shredded coconut, sliced almonds, or any other desired toppings before serving.

Coconut Macaroons

Ingredients:

2 1/2 cups unsweetened shredded coconut

1/2 cup coconut flour

1/2 cup coconut oil, melted

1/2 cup honey or maple syrup

2 teaspoons vanilla extract

Pinch of salt

Optional: Dairy-free chocolate chips or melted dark chocolate for dipping (ensure it's Paleo-friendly)

Instructions:

Preheat your oven to 350°F (175°C). Line a baking sheet with parchment paper.

In a mixing bowl, combine the shredded coconut, coconut flour, melted coconut oil, honey or maple syrup, vanilla extract, and a pinch of salt. Mix until well combined.

Using a cookie scoop or tablespoon, scoop out the mixture and shape it into mounds or small rounds, pressing firmly together to form the macaroons.

Place the formed macaroons onto the lined baking sheet, leaving a bit of space between each one.

Bake in the preheated oven for 12-15 minutes, or until the edges turn golden brown.

Remove from the oven and let the macaroons cool on the baking sheet for a few minutes before transferring them to a wire rack to cool completely.

If desired, melt some dairy-free chocolate chips or dark chocolate in a microwave-safe bowl in 30-second increments, stirring in between until smooth. Dip the cooled macaroons in the melted chocolate or drizzle it over the tops.

Let the chocolate set before serving.

Pumpkin Spice Energy Balls

Ingredients:

1 cup pitted dates, soaked in warm water for 10-15 minutes and drained

1 cup raw cashews

1/2 cup pumpkin puree

1/4 cup unsweetened shredded coconut

1 teaspoon vanilla extract

1 teaspoon ground cinnamon

1/2 teaspoon ground nutmeg

1/4 teaspoon ground ginger

Pinch of ground cloves

Pinch of salt

Additional shredded coconut for rolling (optional)

Instructions:

In a food processor, blend the soaked and drained dates until they form a paste-like consistency.

Add the raw cashews to the food processor and pulse until they are finely chopped and mixed with the date paste.

Add in the pumpkin puree, shredded coconut, vanilla extract, ground cinnamon, ground nutmeg, ground ginger, ground cloves, and a pinch of salt. Process until the mixture forms a dough-like consistency.

Scoop out portions of the mixture and roll them into bite-sized balls using your hands.

Optionally, roll the energy balls in additional shredded coconut to coat the exterior.

Place the energy balls on a plate or tray and refrigerate for at least 30 minutes to allow them to firm up.

Paleo Banana Bread

Ingredients:

4 ripe bananas, mashed

4 eggs

1/2 cup almond butter or cashew butter

1/4 cup coconut oil, melted

1 teaspoon vanilla extract

1/2 cup coconut flour

1 teaspoon baking soda

1 teaspoon ground cinnamon

Pinch of salt

Optional: Chopped nuts, dark chocolate chips, or dried fruits for added texture and flavor

Instructions:

Preheat your oven to 350°F (175°C). Grease or line a loaf pan with parchment paper.

In a large mixing bowl, combine the mashed bananas, eggs, almond butter or cashew butter, melted coconut oil, and vanilla extract. Mix until well combined.

In another bowl, whisk together the coconut flour, baking soda, ground cinnamon, and a pinch of salt.

Gradually add the dry ingredients to the wet ingredients, stirring until thoroughly combined and a smooth batter forms.

Optionally, fold in some chopped nuts, dark chocolate chips, or dried fruits into the batter for extra texture and flavor.

Pour the batter into the prepared loaf pan, spreading it out evenly.

Bake in the preheated oven for 50-60 minutes, or until a toothpick inserted into the center comes out clean.

Once baked, remove the banana bread from the oven and allow it to cool in the pan for 10-15 minutes before transferring it to a wire rack to cool completely.

Chocolate Covered Strawberries

Ingredients:

1 pint fresh strawberries, rinsed and dried

4 ounces Paleo-friendly dark chocolate or dairy-free chocolate chips

1 tablespoon coconut oil

Instructions:

Prepare a baking sheet or plate lined with parchment paper.

In a microwave-safe bowl or using a double boiler, melt the dark chocolate or chocolate chips with the coconut oil. If using a microwave, heat in 30-second intervals, stirring in between until the chocolate is smooth and fully melted.

Hold each strawberry by the stem and dip it into the melted chocolate, swirling to coat it entirely.

Allow any excess chocolate to drip off before placing the chocolate-covered strawberry onto the prepared baking sheet or plate.

Repeat the process with the remaining strawberries until they are all coated with chocolate.

Once all the strawberries are coated, place the baking sheet or plate in the refrigerator for about 15-20 minutes to allow the chocolate to set.

PALEO DIET SOUP RECIPES SOUP

Chicken and Vegetable Soup

Ingredients:

2 tablespoons coconut oil or olive oil

1 onion, diced

3 cloves garlic, minced

2 carrots, peeled and diced

2 celery stalks, diced

1 bell pepper, diced

1 zucchini, diced

1 pound boneless, skinless chicken breasts or thighs, diced

6 cups chicken broth or bone broth

1 can (14 oz) diced tomatoes

1 teaspoon dried thyme

1 teaspoon dried rosemary

Salt and pepper to taste

Chopped fresh parsley for garnish (optional)

Instructions:

In a large pot or Dutch oven, heat the coconut oil or olive oil over medium heat. Add the diced onion and minced garlic. Sauté until the onion becomes translucent.

Add the diced carrots, celery, bell pepper, and zucchini to the pot. Cook for a few minutes, stirring occasionally.

Add the diced chicken to the pot and cook until the chicken is no longer pink.

Pour in the chicken broth and diced tomatoes. Stir well.

Add the dried thyme, dried rosemary, salt, and pepper. Mix everything together.

Bring the soup to a boil, then reduce the heat to low. Cover and simmer for about 20-25 minutes, allowing the flavors to meld and the vegetables to soften.

Taste and adjust the seasoning if needed.

Serve the Paleo chicken and vegetable soup hot, garnished with chopped fresh parsley if desired.

Butternut Squash Soup

Ingredients:

1 medium butternut squash, peeled, seeded, and cubed

1 onion, chopped

2 cloves garlic, minced

2 carrots, peeled and chopped

2 celery stalks, chopped

4 cups chicken or vegetable broth

1 can (13.5 oz) full-fat coconut milk

2 tablespoons coconut oil or olive oil

1 teaspoon ground cinnamon

1/2 teaspoon ground nutmeg

Salt and pepper to taste

Optional toppings: Roasted pumpkin seeds, a drizzle of coconut cream, chopped fresh herbs

Instructions:

In a large pot or Dutch oven, heat the coconut oil or olive oil over medium heat. Add the chopped onion and minced garlic. Sauté until the onion becomes translucent.

Add the chopped carrots and celery to the pot. Cook for a few minutes, stirring occasionally.

Add the cubed butternut squash to the pot and pour in the chicken or vegetable broth.

Bring the mixture to a boil, then reduce the heat to low. Cover and simmer for about 20-25 minutes, or until the butternut squash is tender.

Using an immersion blender or transferring the soup in batches to a blender, blend the soup until smooth and creamy.

Return the blended soup to the pot if needed. Stir in the coconut milk, ground cinnamon, ground nutmeg, salt, and pepper. Mix well.

Simmer the soup for an additional 5-10 minutes to allow the flavors to meld.

Taste and adjust the seasoning if needed.

Serve the Paleo butternut squash soup hot, optionally garnished with roasted pumpkin seeds, a drizzle of coconut cream, or chopped fresh herbs for extra flavor and texture.

Spicy Cauliflower and Cheddar Soup

Ingredients:

1 head cauliflower, chopped into florets

1 onion, diced

2 cloves garlic, minced

4 cups vegetable or chicken broth

1 cup sharp cheddar cheese, shredded

1/2 cup heavy cream

2 tablespoons olive oil

1 teaspoon paprika

1/2 teaspoon cayenne pepper (adjust to taste)

Salt and pepper to taste

Optional: Chopped green onions for garnish

Instructions:

In a large pot, heat olive oil over medium heat. Add diced onion and minced garlic, sauté until onions are translucent.

Add cauliflower florets to the pot and sauté for a few minutes.

Pour in the vegetable or chicken broth, covering the cauliflower. Bring to a boil, then reduce heat and simmer for about 15-20 minutes or until the cauliflower is tender.

Use an immersion blender or transfer the mixture to a blender to puree until smooth.

Return the pureed soup to the pot over low heat. Stir in the heavy cream, shredded cheddar cheese, paprika, and cayenne pepper.

Let the soup simmer for an additional 5-10 minutes, stirring occasionally until the cheese melts and the soup thickens.

Season with salt and pepper to taste.

Serve the soup hot, garnished with chopped green onions if desired.

Turkey and Vegetable Soup

Ingredients:

1 lb ground turkey

1 onion, chopped

2 carrots, diced

2 celery stalks, diced

2 cloves garlic, minced

4 cups chicken or vegetable broth

1 can (14 oz) diced tomatoes

1 teaspoon dried thyme

1 teaspoon dried oregano

Salt and pepper to taste

Fresh parsley for garnish (optional)

Instructions:

In a large pot, cook the ground turkey over medium heat until browned. Drain any excess fat and set aside.

In the same pot, add chopped onion, diced carrots, diced celery, and minced garlic. Sauté until the vegetables are tender.

Add the cooked turkey back to the pot along with the chicken or vegetable broth, diced tomatoes (with their juices), dried thyme, and dried oregano.

Bring the mixture to a boil, then reduce heat and simmer for about 15-20 minutes to allow the flavors to blend.

Season with salt and pepper to taste.

Serve the soup hot, garnished with fresh parsley if desired.

Creamy Broccoli and Cheese Soup

Ingredients:

4 cups fresh broccoli florets

1 onion, chopped

2 cloves garlic, minced

4 cups chicken or vegetable broth

1 cup heavy cream

2 cups shredded cheddar cheese

2 tablespoons butter

Salt and pepper to taste

Optional: Crispy bacon bits for garnish

Instructions:

In a large pot, melt butter over medium heat. Add chopped onion and minced garlic, sauté until softened and fragrant.

Add broccoli florets to the pot and sauté for a few minutes until they begin to soften.

Pour in the chicken or vegetable broth, covering the broccoli. Bring to a boil, then reduce heat and simmer for about 10-15 minutes until the broccoli is tender.

Use an immersion blender or transfer the mixture to a blender to puree until smooth.

Return the pureed soup to the pot over low heat. Stir in the heavy cream and shredded cheddar cheese, allowing the cheese to melt into the soup.

Season with salt and pepper to taste.

Serve the soup hot, optionally garnished with crispy bacon bits for added flavor.

Mexican Chicken and Cauliflower Rice Soup

Ingredients:

1 lb boneless, skinless chicken breasts, diced

1 onion, chopped

2 cloves garlic, minced

4 cups chicken broth

1 can (14 oz) diced tomatoes with green chilies

2 cups cauliflower rice

1 teaspoon cumin

1 teaspoon chili powder

Salt and pepper to taste

Fresh cilantro for garnish (optional)

Lime wedges for serving (optional)

Instructions:

In a large pot, heat a bit of oil over medium heat. Add diced chicken and cook until browned and cooked through. Remove from the pot and set aside.

In the same pot, add chopped onion and sauté until translucent. Add minced garlic and cook for another minute.

Pour in the chicken broth, diced tomatoes with green chilies (undrained), and cauliflower rice. Bring to a simmer.

Stir in the cooked chicken, cumin, and chili powder. Simmer for about 15-20 minutes.

Season with salt and pepper to taste.

Serve the soup hot, garnished with fresh cilantro and a lime wedge if desired.

Creamy Spinach and Artichoke Soup

Ingredients:

2 cups fresh spinach leaves, chopped

1 can (14 oz) artichoke hearts, drained and chopped

1 onion, chopped

2 cloves garlic, minced

4 cups chicken or vegetable broth

1 cup heavy cream

1 cup shredded mozzarella cheese

2 tablespoons butter

Salt and pepper to taste

Optional: Grated Parmesan cheese for garnish

Instructions:

In a large pot, melt butter over medium heat. Add chopped onion and minced garlic, sauté until softened and fragrant.

Add chopped spinach and chopped artichoke hearts to the pot. Cook for a few minutes until spinach wilts.

Pour in the chicken or vegetable broth and bring to a simmer. Let it cook for about 10-15 minutes.

Stir in the heavy cream and shredded mozzarella cheese, allowing the cheese to melt into the soup.

Continue to simmer for an additional 5-10 minutes, stirring occasionally.

Season with salt and pepper to taste.

Serve the soup hot, optionally garnished with grated Parmesan cheese for added flavor.

Creamy Tomato Basil Soup

Ingredients:

4 cups fresh tomatoes, chopped

1 onion, chopped

2 cloves garlic, minced

4 cups vegetable or chicken broth

1/2 cup heavy cream

1/4 cup fresh basil leaves, chopped

2 tablespoons olive oil

Salt and pepper to taste

Optional: Fresh basil leaves for garnish

Instructions:

In a large pot, heat olive oil over medium heat. Add chopped onion and minced garlic, sauté until onions are translucent.

Add chopped tomatoes to the pot and cook for about 5-7 minutes until they begin to soften.

Pour in the vegetable or chicken broth, covering the tomatoes and onions. Bring to a boil, then reduce heat and simmer for about 15-20 minutes.

Use an immersion blender or transfer the mixture to a blender to puree until smooth.

Return the pureed soup to the pot over low heat. Stir in the heavy cream and chopped fresh basil.

Season with salt and pepper to taste.

Simmer the soup for an additional 5-10 minutes, allowing the flavors to meld together.

Serve the soup hot, optionally garnished with fresh basil leaves.

Broccoli and Bacon Soup

Ingredients:

4 slices bacon, chopped

1 onion, diced

3 cloves garlic, minced

4 cups broccoli florets

3 cups chicken or vegetable broth

1 cup full-fat coconut milk

Salt and pepper to taste

Optional toppings: Chopped green onions, crispy bacon bits

Instructions:

In a large pot or Dutch oven, cook the chopped bacon over medium heat until crispy. Remove the crispy bacon bits and set them aside for later, leaving the bacon grease in the pot.

In the same pot with the bacon grease, add the diced onion and minced garlic. Sauté until the onion becomes translucent.

Add the broccoli florets to the pot and stir to combine with the onions and garlic.

Pour in the chicken or vegetable broth. Bring the mixture to a boil, then reduce the heat to low. Cover and simmer for about 15-20 minutes, or until the broccoli is tender.

Using an immersion blender or transferring the soup in batches to a blender, blend the soup until smooth.

Return the blended soup to the pot if needed. Stir in the coconut milk and mix well.

Simmer the soup for an additional 5-10 minutes to heat through and meld the flavors.

Season with salt and pepper to taste.

Serve the Paleo broccoli and bacon soup hot, garnished with the reserved crispy bacon bits and chopped green onions if desired.

Sweet Potato and Coconut Soup

Ingredients:

2 tablespoons coconut oil

1 onion, diced

2 cloves garlic, minced

2 large sweet potatoes, peeled and diced

4 cups vegetable or chicken broth

1 can (14 oz) full-fat coconut milk

1 teaspoon ground cumin

1/2 teaspoon ground coriander

Pinch of cayenne pepper (optional, for heat)

Salt and pepper to taste

Fresh cilantro for garnish (optional)

Instructions:

In a large pot, heat the coconut oil over medium heat. Add the diced onion and minced garlic. Sauté until the onion turns soft and translucent.

Add the diced sweet potatoes to the pot and stir to combine with the onions and garlic.

Pour in the vegetable or chicken broth. Bring the mixture to a boil, then reduce the heat to low. Cover and simmer for about 15-20 minutes, or until the sweet potatoes are tender.

Using an immersion blender or transferring the soup in batches to a blender, blend the soup until smooth and creamy.

Return the blended soup to the pot if needed. Stir in the coconut milk, ground cumin, ground coriander, cayenne pepper (if using), salt, and pepper. Mix well to combine.

Simmer the soup for an additional 5-10 minutes to allow the flavors to meld.

Taste and adjust the seasoning if needed.

Serve the Paleo sweet potato and coconut soup hot, optionally garnished with fresh cilantro for extra flavor.

Paleo Chicken and Kale Soup

Ingredients:

1 tablespoon olive oil or coconut oil

1 onion, diced

2 cloves garlic, minced

2 carrots, sliced

2 celery stalks, sliced

1 pound boneless, skinless chicken thighs or breasts, diced

6 cups chicken broth or bone broth

1 can (14 oz) diced tomatoes

1 teaspoon dried thyme

1 teaspoon dried oregano

4 cups chopped kale leaves, stems removed

Salt and pepper to taste

Chopped fresh parsley for garnish (optional)

Instructions:

In a large pot or Dutch oven, heat the olive oil or coconut oil over medium heat. Add the diced onion and minced garlic. Sauté until the onion becomes translucent.

Add the sliced carrots and celery to the pot. Cook for a few minutes, stirring occasionally.

Add the diced chicken to the pot and cook until it's no longer pink.

Pour in the chicken broth and diced tomatoes (with their juices). Stir well to combine.

Add the dried thyme, dried oregano, salt, and pepper. Mix everything together.

Bring the soup to a boil, then reduce the heat to low. Cover and simmer for about 15-20 minutes.

Add the chopped kale to the pot and simmer for an additional 5-10 minutes, or until the kale is wilted and tender.

Taste and adjust the seasoning if needed.

Serve the Paleo chicken and kale soup hot, optionally garnished with chopped fresh parsley for extra flavor.

Tomato Basil Soup

Ingredients:

2 tablespoons olive oil

1 onion, chopped

3 cloves garlic, minced

1 can (28 oz) diced tomatoes

2 cups chicken or vegetable broth

1/4 cup fresh basil leaves, chopped (plus extra for garnish)

1 teaspoon dried oregano

Salt and pepper to taste

Optional: Coconut cream for garnish

Instructions:

In a large pot, heat the olive oil over medium heat. Add the chopped onion and minced garlic. Sauté until the onion becomes translucent.

Add the diced tomatoes (with their juices) to the pot. Stir and cook for a few minutes.

Pour in the chicken or vegetable broth. Add the chopped basil leaves and dried oregano. Stir well to combine.

Bring the mixture to a boil, then reduce the heat to low. Cover and simmer for about 15-20 minutes to allow the flavors to meld.

Using an immersion blender or transferring the soup in batches to a blender, blend the soup until smooth and creamy.

Return the blended soup to the pot if needed. Season with salt and pepper to taste, adjusting the seasoning as desired.

Serve the Paleo tomato basil soup hot, garnished with extra fresh basil leaves and a drizzle of coconut cream if desired.

Zucchini and Carrot Soup

Ingredients:

2 tablespoons olive oil or coconut oil

1 onion, chopped

2 cloves garlic, minced

4 medium zucchinis, chopped

3 large carrots, peeled and chopped

4 cups vegetable or chicken broth

1 teaspoon dried thyme

1 teaspoon dried basil

Salt and pepper to taste

Chopped fresh parsley for garnish (optional)

Instructions:

In a large pot or Dutch oven, heat the olive oil or coconut oil over medium heat. Add the chopped onion and minced garlic. Sauté until the onion becomes translucent.

Add the chopped zucchinis and carrots to the pot. Cook for a few minutes, stirring occasionally.

Pour in the vegetable or chicken broth. Add the dried thyme, dried basil, salt, and pepper. Stir well to combine.

Bring the mixture to a boil, then reduce the heat to low. Cover and simmer for about 15-20 minutes, or until the zucchinis and carrots are tender.

Using an immersion blender or transferring the soup in batches to a blender, blend the soup until smooth and creamy.

Return the blended soup to the pot if needed. Taste and adjust the seasoning if needed.

Serve the Paleo zucchini and carrot soup hot, optionally garnished with chopped fresh parsley for extra flavor.

Mushroom and Spinach Soup

Ingredients:

2 tablespoons ghee or coconut oil

1 onion, diced

3 cloves garlic, minced

8 ounces cremini or button mushrooms, sliced

6 cups chicken or vegetable broth

4 cups fresh spinach leaves

1 teaspoon dried thyme

1 teaspoon dried rosemary

Salt and pepper to taste

Optional: Coconut cream for garnish

Instructions:

In a large pot or Dutch oven, heat the ghee or coconut oil over medium heat. Add the diced onion and minced garlic. Sauté until the onion becomes translucent.

Add the sliced mushrooms to the pot. Cook for a few minutes until the mushrooms begin to soften and release their juices.

Pour in the chicken or vegetable broth. Add the dried thyme, dried rosemary, salt, and pepper. Stir well to combine.

Bring the soup to a gentle boil, then reduce the heat to low. Cover and simmer for about 15-20 minutes, allowing the flavors to meld.

Add the fresh spinach leaves to the pot and simmer for an additional 3-5 minutes until the spinach wilts.

Taste and adjust the seasoning if needed.

Serve the Paleo mushroom and spinach soup hot, optionally garnishing each bowl with a drizzle of coconut cream for extra richness.

Chicken and Coconut Curry Soup

Ingredients:

1 tablespoon coconut oil

1 onion, diced

3 cloves garlic, minced

1 tablespoon grated ginger

1 pound boneless, skinless chicken breasts or thighs, cut into cubes

2 tablespoons curry powder

1 can (14 oz) full-fat coconut milk

4 cups chicken broth

2 cups chopped vegetables (bell peppers, carrots, broccoli, etc.)

Salt and pepper to taste

Chopped cilantro for garnish (optional)

Instructions:

In a large pot, heat the coconut oil over medium heat. Add the diced onion, minced garlic, and grated ginger. Sauté until the onion becomes translucent and fragrant.

Add the cubed chicken to the pot. Cook until the chicken is no longer pink.

Sprinkle the curry powder over the chicken and onion mixture. Stir well to coat the chicken with the curry powder.

Pour in the coconut milk and chicken broth. Stir to combine.

Add the chopped vegetables to the pot. Bring the soup to a simmer and cook for about 15-20 minutes, or until the vegetables are tender.

Season the soup with salt and pepper to taste.

Serve the Paleo chicken and coconut curry soup hot, optionally garnished with chopped cilantro for extra flavor.

CHAPTER 7: SUSTAINABILITY AND LONG-TERM LIFESTYLE INTEGRATION

Everyone has their own opinion on whether or not the Paleo Diet can be maintained over the long run. Although the diet promotes nutrient-dense whole foods and discourages processed foods, some people may find it difficult to adhere to the severe rules of the diet, especially the elimination of whole food categories such as grains, legumes, and dairy.

How feasible it is to stick to the diet in different cultural, social, and lifestyle settings is one factor to think about. When going out to restaurants, going to parties, or traveling, it might be difficult to stick to the Paleo Diet because there may not be many Paleo-friendly options. A sense of limitation or loneliness may result, which may affect long-term commitment.

Furthermore, if not properly planned, the elimination of specific food categories might lead to worries about possible nutritional shortages. For instance, cutting out grains might mean less of a supply of fiber and several vitamins that are naturally present in whole grains. Similarly, if you don't eat dairy, you could not get enough calcium and vitamin D from your diet or from supplements.

Modesty and adaptability are key to making the Paleo Diet work for you in the long run. A more flexible interpretation of the Paleo Diet that permits the occasional exception or reintroduction of specific foods according to individual tolerance may be more suitable for some people's lifestyles while still adhering to the diet's principals.

Personal choices and medical requirements are another factor to think about. The Paleo Diet may not be right for everyone, even though its principles do help some people achieve their health goals. A more well-rounded diet that allows for additional grains, legumes, and dairy products without negatively impacting health may be more appealing to some.

Individual preferences, health objectives, cultural influences, and practical considerations are the most important elements in determining the long-term viability of dietary choices. The Paleo Diet provides a foundation based on whole foods and evolutionary thinking, but it may need personal adjustments, moderation, and adaptability to fit different lifestyle variables and tastes if it is to be sustainable in the long run. To find out how to incorporate Paleo Diet principles into a sustainable lifestyle that fits one's health needs and objectives in the long run, it might be helpful to consult with healthcare providers or certified dietitians.

Creating Sustainable Habits

Integrating Paleo Diet concepts into everyday activities in a reasonable and pleasurable way is key to creating sustainable habits within this framework. In order to form habits that will last, it is important to start small and create attainable goals. Make gradual, manageable adjustments to your food and lifestyle that are in line with the Paleo

Diet's principals rather than trying to make a complete overhaul all at once.

Preparing meals in advance is essential for sticking to the Paleo Diet. Making it a practice to plan meals ahead of time, buy authorized items in bulk, and prepare meals for the week ahead of time makes it much easier to have selections that are compliant on hand. A great way to make sticking to the Paleo diet easier is to prepare meals in bulk and store them in portions so you can grab one while you're on the go.

A vital part of sustainability is learning about Paleo-friendly dishes and trying them out. To make the Paleo diet more manageable in the long term, it's a good idea to try new recipes often, find tasty alternatives to limited foods, and modify old favorites to fit the plan. Creating a collection of healthy and delicious Paleo recipes that you can rely on might help you stick to your eating plan.

Adaptability and the freedom to make little changes here and there to meet personal tastes are key to long-term viability. Maintaining adherence to the Paleo Diet principles while allowing for occasional treats or adjustments according to individual tolerance or social circumstances might help keep the diet more manageable in the long run by avoiding feelings of restriction or deprivation.

Building durable habits requires consistency and persistence. Be patient and dedicated if you want to make the Paleo Diet your way of life. Mindful eating habits are more likely to last in the long run when practiced regularly and in accordance with the diet's principles.

In addition, the Paleo Diet is best followed loosely as an outline rather than a bible. Diets are more likely to be sustainable when they are adaptable to the demands of their participants, when they are willing to try new things and are willing to make adjustments as they go. Building long-term habits on the Paleo Diet requires consistent self-evaluation and dietary adjustments to meet changing lifestyle requirements. Seeking advice from healthcare providers or certified dietitians can provide valuable help in developing long-term habits that are in line with personal health objectives and preferences.

Adapting Paleo into Everyday Life

Making the Paleo Diet work for you means finding realistic and long-term ways to incorporate its ideas into your daily life. Meal planning and grocery buying are important parts. To create a Paleo-friendly kitchen, make it a habit to choose lean meats, a variety of fresh fruits and vegetables, nuts, seeds, and healthy fats, and cut out processed and refined meals. Making a Paleo Diet-compliant shopping list and basing meal plans on these categories will help you stay on track and make sure you have all the authorized foods on hand.

If you want to follow the Paleo Diet consistently, you need to start prepping your meals. Making Paleo-friendly dishes at home on a regular basis is a great way to stick to the diet. To fit hectic schedules and reduce dependence on non-compliant foods, this practice could entail meal preparing, bulk cooking, or meal planning in advance.

The Paleo Diet may be easily integrated into daily life by being careful of food choices while eating out or spending time with friends and family. Even when you're not at home, you can still stick to the diet's principals by eating lean meats, veggies, and healthy fats in simpler recipes and eliminating grains, legumes, and dairy.

Making the Paleo Diet a regular part of your life is easier with the help of a supportive community and open lines of communication with loved ones. If you want to make it simpler to keep to your diet in different social circumstances, sharing your dietary preferences or requirements with friends, family, or coworkers may help establish understanding and support.

Another thing that might help with sticking to the Paleo Diet is being flexible and letting yourself make the odd mistake without ruining the whole program. Diets are more likely to be successful in the long run when participants accept that perfection is unattainable and are willing to make adjustments when needed or for special occasions.

Last but not least, the Paleo Diet can be more easily integrated into daily life if its concept is accepted as a framework rather than a rigid set of regulations. Integrating the Paleo Diet into one's daily routine may be made more sustainable and practical by acknowledging that it can be adjusted to fit one's preferences and requirements while staying true to its fundamental principles. For tailored advice on how to successfully incorporate Paleo Diet principles into daily life, taking into account specific health objectives and dietary restrictions, it is recommended to consult with healthcare providers or certified dietitians.